MW01235203

Chasing Fireflies
Paige P. Horne

Dedication: To all those who suffer in silence. You matter.

Sheila,

Thank you for our talks and your support!

Love
Paige P. Horne

A note from the author:

Depression is not something to take lightly. If you or someone you know is suffering with this illness, please reach out and call the National Suicide Prevention Lifeline at 1-800-273-8255. Also, you can text the Crisis Text Line if you need someone to talk to in a non-life-threatening crisis by texting START to 741-741. Never lose your hope. People often don't understand suicide, and I've heard it being called selfish. I have mixed feelings with it now after all the research I've done. Two people close to me chose to take their own life, and at first I was angry and of course hurt, but I now realize they were hurting deeper than people without depression can fully understand.

Published: Paige P. Horne 2016

Pgpeacock13@gmail.com

Editor: Paige Maroney Smith

Cover design: designs@pinkinkdesigns.com

Proofreaders: Crystal Jones, Monica Lewis, Julie T.

Prologue

Present Day

Cash

I lift my head off of the steering wheel and look out my windshield. My mind is foggy, and I can't seem to wrap my brain around reality. Rain falls heavy outside and beats against the old truck's metal roof. We've lived in this town for eight years now, and somehow it doesn't feel like home anymore. I wipe my eyes and open Old Blue's door. I'd like to say I've never been here before, but that's a lie I can't tell. I step out onto ground I've stepped onto more times than I can count, but for better reasons. I'm losing my mind, and I've lost my crazy heart. The rain soaks me, but like the inside, my outside is numb, too. Music flows through the opened door of the small-town bar, and like a zombie, I walk inside. Sweet guitar strings are strummed, but all I hear is the ringing in my ears. I take a seat on the barstool as Banner walks over.

"Heavy rain tonight," he says, sliding a napkin in front of me. I look at the napkin and then up at his face.

"Jack—straight up."

He narrows his eyes, but doesn't question me. I watch him as he reaches up to grab a shot glass. Looking down at my hands, I run a finger over the dried blood that covers my palm. Water drops from the tip of my baseball hat, and my eyes shut for a brief moment. Memories flood my mind––blonde curls and baby blue eyes. Painful moments and a lifetime of struggles, but I'd do it all again. I open my eyes and grab the glass in front of me. I toss back the burning liquid and try not to choke on the sadness that threatens to take my life away.

I put the glass down and look up when Banner asks, "Another?" I nod and my hand shakes as I bring it to my greedy mouth. "You okay, Cash? Can I get you anything else?" His concern slips between his lips, and my whole body starts to shake. I look up from my shot glass.

"Stolen time," I whisper as my eyes cast downward, and my heart falters.

Chapter One

Our Wedding Day. Eight Years Earlier.

Cash

I lean against the hotel bedroom door and watch as she looks at herself in the mirror. Her eyes meet mine, and I see it when her cheeks turn a pretty shade of pink.

"You're perfect."

"You're only saying that because I married you."

"I'm saying that because it's true," I say, shutting the door behind me. I set the bucket of ice down and walk over to her. She's in a cream-colored lace dress and has a flower in her wild curly hair. We just tied the knot. We dated throughout high school, and four years after graduation, I finally asked her to be mine for life. She agreed, and after a long engagement, we took a trip to the courthouse. With only a few people to witness, we promised each other forever. Wrapping my arms around her waist, I kiss her dirty blonde curls and she rocks us from side to side.

"Why can't I be happy all the time?" she whispers to me, like it's a secret. But in a way, it is. Sometimes it's hard for the girl I love to get out of bed, and there are times that she only does it for me. But there are also times when I'm not even enough to fight the darkness away.

I kiss her again and tell her once more, "You're perfect. You're enough. You're mine." She gives me her smile, and I turn her around to face me. I look into her pretty blue eyes and see my soul. It reflects within her and I think, *how lucky am I to find someone like this?* I see how much she loves me through her eyes, and I hope she can see it through mine, too.

I kiss her lips, and she removes my blazer. Our sweet love turns into needy love, and I lift her up and place her onto the dresser, knocking over the bucket of ice I got only minutes before. We ignore it, and I grip onto her thighs as she runs her fingers up the back of my neck and into my hair, causing chills to cover my body as I kiss her crazy. I lift her dress, and she undoes my belt and pants. Within minutes, I'm where I want to be, and she's closing her eyes. I move and she wraps her thighs around my waist tighter as I lay her down onto the bed. My wife's hands go to the pillows above us, and she grips tight as I show her how much I love her. I tell her, too, as I kiss down her neck and grip onto her hips. Pulling her closer to me and pushing down deeper, I make us whole, and she makes my world brighter. I kiss her again, and when I pull away, wild love tells me how happy I make her. Time gives you the kind of love we have, and I pray for more of it every day as I watch her come undone underneath me.

Chapter Two
Five Year Anniversary
Cash

"This house is everything!" my wife yells as she twirls around on the front porch. I watch her with absolute amazement.

"Be careful, baby. Some of these boards don't look so great," I say. She giggles and runs inside. I adjust the box in my hand and follow, shaking my head at my crazy wife. The sound of her running bounces off the old walls of the big farmhouse, and I set the box down by the front door. Taking a look around, I can't help but smile. We're finally here. The house has been around since the twenties, and the field that surrounds it used to be alive—nothing but dead wheat grass now and a bur oak tree that's seen many years before us, but she doesn't care and neither do I. After years of saving up and months of looking, we finally found a place. We went to the bank, put down everything we had, and got a loan big enough so we could have extra to fix her up. I hear the creaky springs of our used mattress, and I make my way up the stairs.

Her laugh is the only sound I want to follow, and I smile when I see her jumping on our bed. She falls on her back, and I lean against the doorway, watching her.

"Cash, I'm so happy." She turns to look at me and smiles. Her eyes sparkle with light as the sun shines through the windows of our bedroom, making her hair look golden blonde.

"You are?"

"Yes."

I push off the wall and walk over to her. "How happy?" I ask, looking down at her spread-out curls. She stretches her arms wide, showing me how much. She closes her eyes, and at the same time, I lean down quickly, tickling her crazy until she can't breathe and complains her ribs ache. I kiss them better, and my hand crawls up her skirt. She lets me do what I want and I do. I take her face in my hands and kiss her mouth. She tugs my shirt loose from my pants and pulls it up and over my head. My lips touch her neck and make their way down to her collarbone. She breathes heavy and reaches for my belt. After she slides it through the loops, she tosses it and unbuttons my pants. I tug them down and hike her summertime dress up. My fingers dig into her thighs, and within seconds I'm inside her. Pushing and pulling. Taking and giving. She's everything to me, and I'm her fucking lifeline.

*

The moving crew finished bringing everything in earlier this afternoon, so we sit at the kitchen table eating cold ham sandwiches with salt and vinegar potato chips for supper because we didn't feel like going grocery shopping just yet. The countertops are filled with stacked dishes and glasses that need to be put away still, and the rest of the house is equally a mess, but there's plenty of time to get to it.

"The lights get cut on tomorrow," I tell her as she strikes a match and holds it to the candlewick.

"I like it better this way." She smiles and the fifty candles in the small room reflect off of her pretty face. She sits and I jump up, remembering it's not only move-in day but also our anniversary.

"Where are you going?" she asks.

"I'll be right back." I grab the bouquet of roses out of the small closet in the living room I bought for her earlier today and hide them behind my back. She narrows her eyes at me when I walk back in.

"What you got back there?"

I walk over to her and lay the flowers down onto the table. She smiles and I grab her chair after I sit and bring it and her closer to me. I look at her face and down at her lips.

"Happy anniversary, baby." I kiss her lips, and she grabs the flowers and brings them to her face.

"They smell pretty."

"They smell pretty?" I ask. "How does something smell pretty?"

She shrugs. "They just do."

"You smell pretty." I grin.

We eat in silence until we hear a squeaking noise. Our eyes lock. Hers are filled with wonder and slight fear. Mine are filled with dread.

"Mice," I say.

"We have to get some traps. But don't you let me see one on there." She puts a chip into her mouth and nearly spits it out when a mouse runs across the floor. "Holy shit." She coughs and pulls her feet up. I pat her back.

"You aren't scared of a little mouse, are you?"

"Yes! It might get my toes."

I lean down and kiss her big toe. “Nothing is going to get your toes, woman.” I’m given another giggle, but she keeps her feet up for the rest of supper.

*

I sit on our bed and look out the bare windows in our bedroom. The moon shines through leaving a trail of light across our wooden floors, and I can see the tree outside shift from the wind.

“I’ll go into town tomorrow and get some traps. You want to ride with me?” I ask, still looking out the window. Hearing no answer, I turn as she walks out of the bathroom, mindlessly rubbing lotion on her hands.

“Sara,” I say, getting her attention. She looks up, and I can see it. That blank stare—that I’m-fading-into-a-different-mindset look in her soft blue eyes. The mattress dips when she sits down, and I run my finger over her hand. “Baby, I’m going into town tomorrow. Come with me.”

“I may not feel up to it.” She lifts her feet from the floor and lies down. I rub my face and look over at her as she grabs the covers and pulls them up to her chin. I look back down at the moonlight and wonder if the covers make her feel safe or if it’s something more. Getting up, I lean down and blow the candles out. I remove my T-shirt and lift the covers to get into bed. Lying down, I grab her by her waist and pull her to my side. Wrapping my arms around her, I put my face into her neck and breathe her in. I don't want the damn covers to make her feel safe. I want to make her feel that way.

"You'll feel better tomorrow," I murmur against her soft skin.

"We'll see," she says.

"Yeah," I agree quietly. "I'll love you forever."

"Forever is such a long time," she replies. "You'll get tired of me."

"Never," I say. She sighs and I don't fall asleep until I feel her breathing even out.

*

The old truck my dad shockingly handed down to me years ago backfires and Sara thinks it's funny today. We call him Old Blue, and that's exactly what he is—old and blue. He's a smelly 1971 Ford, makes a funny noise when you press the gas, and the heat doesn't work, but he's ours. Old Blue is paid for and gets us where we need to go. Sara laughs when I hit the gas pedal, and he makes a loud popping sound, but then she gets mad because the rusted floorboard is hot against her bare feet.

"You should put your sandals back on," I tell her.

"I don't like shoes," she says. I roll my eyes.

"I saw that." She smacks my arm, and I try not to smile.

"You complain too much," I say, looking over at her piled-up curls. She wears a short summer dress that says something about Woodstock, peace, and love.

"Oh, yeah?" She lifts her brow and pokes her lips out at me.

"Absolutely," I confirm. She lifts her feet and slides across the bench seat, moving closer.

"What are you doing?" I ask as she leans into the crook of my neck, and I feel her sweet breath against my skin.

"Nothing," she whispers into my ear before I feel her tongue running along the side. I move my head away. "I don't think so." She puts her hand on the other side of my face and presses it closer to her. She spreads kisses down to my collarbone and laughs lightly.

"Sara," I breathe out because her other hand is rubbing at the crotch of my jeans. She sucks on my skin and lets out a noise that goes straight to my hardness. "Baby," I say as she keeps kissing and sucking. My eyes grow lazy, and my foot gets heavy on the gas. I don't even notice that we pass by a cop, but I do when I see blue lights. "Shit. Baby, get back to your side." She laughs as she hurries to her side of the truck. I pull over and wait for the cop to get out. She stifles a laugh as he makes it up to the door, and I shake my head at her as she puts her hand over her mouth and clears her throat. Her eyes look down at my jeans, and I adjust myself before I look over when the cop taps on the glass, signaling for me to roll the window down. It takes a minute because the damn handle needs some grease.

I clear my throat. "How can I help you, officer?"

"Son, do you know you were speeding back there?"

"I didn't realize it," I answer. He looks over at my wife, and I see his eyes move downward. I look over, too. Her dress is riding up from where she moved so quickly. She notices and tugs it down. She sucks her lips in, and her cheeks turn pink. Looking back at the cop, I see he is the chief.

"Okay, you two. How about we pay better attention to driving when we are on the road and less on…" He clears his throat. "Less on each other."

"Yes, sir," I reply.

"You folks have a nice day." He tilts his hat, and as he turns to walk away, I get an idea.

"Hey, chief," I say, sticking my head out the window and looking back at him.

"Yes, son?"

"You doing any hiring?"

He looks me over for a moment and then asks, "You got any experience?"

"Worked under my dad one town over since I was sixteen," I say. "He's been the sheriff for going on thirty years."

He nods in approval. "Well, you come on down to the office tomorrow then. We'll see what we can do."

"Thank you." I smile before I turn back to Sara. She has a look of disappointment on her face, and I sigh inwardly, waiting for the battle I know is coming. I grab the gear shifter and put the truck in drive before pressing the gas.

"You're leaving me," she pouts.

"Baby, please don't start this."

"Oh, I'm starting?" she says sarcastically. She's really pissed, but I can't do anything about it.

"Yes, you are. I have to work."

"No, you don't. We can get by with my disability check and savings for a little while."

"No, we can't, Sara. We don't have any savings. We only have money to fix up that house. You know I have to work."

"You just want to leave me. I'm too much for you, and you can't deal with me all of the time. Just tell me, Cash. Tell me the truth."

"Stop this bullshit, now, Sara," I say, pulling into town. She huffs, and I shake my head when she crosses her arms and looks out her window. We pass by the small-town square with a white gazebo in the middle and sidewalks leading in different directions. Beds of flowers are laid out in different areas, and people are walking everywhere. I notice a few small shops, and I see a sign that reads *Chief's Office*. I park the truck in front of the hardware store and look over at my pouting wife. "You coming in with me?"

"Well, I'm sure you can go in by yourself. Since you need time away from me."

"I don't want to go in by myself." She looks away. I reach over and tug her arm. Yanking it away, she moves as far from me as she can.

"Sara."

"Just go in without me, Cash."

I put the truck in park and kill the engine. Moving closer to her, I softly kiss her neck and feel her restraint melting away. "Please walk inside with me," I ask sweetly. I feel it when she shivers, and I see the goose bumps run across her soft skin.

"Fine," she huffs. "You've given me gooses." She tries to play mad, but I see her smile as she opens her door. And just to see her smile more, I get out on her side, too.

*

I pull her along as I look at the signs above the aisles, trying to find mousetraps—the sticky kind, because Sara doesn't want the old-fashioned ones.

"Oh, Cash, look," she says, dragging me away from the aisle we need to go down. "I've always wanted a hat like this." It's a green floppy hat. Sara puts it on and grins at me.

"Get it," I tell her. She looks at the tag.

"They want too much."

"Just get it."

She scrunches her nose and puts her lips together as she thinks on it for a minute. I grin at her.

"It's not a life-changing decision, woman."

She looks up at me before she shrugs. "I guess I'll get it."

I grab her hand. "Come on. Let's grab some mousetraps, and then I need to go look at the lumber for our porch."

*

"Thanks, man."

"No problem. You new in town?" the man who looks a year or two older than me asks as he helps me put my supplies in the back of Old Blue. He removes his gloves, lifts his hat, and runs a hand through his dark hair.

"Yeah, my wife and I just moved here. Bought that old farmhouse on Eighteenth."

"Damn, that place has been empty for a while."

"We can tell." I laugh.

"Well, it's nice to meet you. Name's Mark Phillips." He places his hat back on his head and reaches to shake my hand. "Let me know if you need any help with the repairs. I learned a thing or two working here."

"Thanks. I'm Cash Williams, and I may take you up on that. My wife isn't too great with a hammer." I smile.

"Hey, I heard that," she says, walking toward us with her floppy hat on and two melting ice cream cones.

"It isn't a secret, baby."

She hands me the cone and rolls her eyes. "Hi, I'm Sara," she says, moving to hold out her hand, but there is ice cream on it, so she takes it back.

"Sorry. Sticky fingers."

Mark laughs. "Nice to meet you. I'm Mark. You two should come over for supper sometime. My wife, Leigh, tells me I cook a mean grilled steak." He winks.

"We may do that," I say. "Appreciate your help." I walk around the truck and open the door for Sara to climb in. Once I get in, too, I start Old Blue and put her in drive.

"He seemed nice," she says, licking her vanilla ice cream.

"Yeah," I agree.

"Let's grab some groceries and then head back home."

*

After we get all of our shopping done, we leave town and turn back onto our road. "I think I'm going to like it here." I look over at my wife and out at the vast land that surrounds us. It's secluded out our way—nothing but fields and woods. I see our house come into view, and I slow the truck down. We have a circular driveway and an old barn at the rear of the house. Nothing else but wheat fields in the back and across the road from us. Our front porch is big enough for some rocking chairs, and it already holds a swing, but it's got some boards that need replacing, so that's what I'm going to work on in the next day or so. I stop the truck, and we climb out. I grab the boards I bought from the back and walk them to the porch before we head inside to get ready for supper.

*

"I could get used to this view," my wife says. I grin and look down. I'm shirtless, screwing in a light bulb on our front porch for when the power gets cut on. It's nice out, and a breeze blows in from the wheat field. Sara sits on the porch swing, one knee bent and the other lightly kicking off of the porch. Her baby pink toes hardly touch the ground, but she makes it work.

"Well, you'll be seeing a lot of it." I climb down from the ladder and fold it together. "This house needs a ton of work."

"I can help, you know."

"I'll put you to work then, woman."

"We'll be coworkers." She winks. I take a seat beside her, and she lifts her other leg up, letting me push us now.

"I do believe you're the prettiest coworker I've ever had."

Her lips lift. "You're only saying that because I married you."

"I'm saying it because it's true."

Shaking her head slightly, she hugs her knees and looks out into the yard.

"Do you want babies?" she asks after a minute.

"I want whatever you want."

"What if our babies have my disorder?"

"We'll deal. Like we deal now," I tell her. She grabs my hand and lightly runs her fingers over my palm.

"You have rough hands." She laces our fingers together. "Our hands don't fit."

"They fit perfect." I hold hers tighter and bring it to my lips, lightly kissing each of her fingers before I put our hands back down.

"Why do you love me so much?" she asks. I look up and push off of the porch. The old swing creaks as I think about her question.

"My love for you makes me who I am. Without it I'd be a different person. Just as the ocean would be different without the waves, the blue sky without the sun, the darkness without the light. You are my other half. You are what makes me… me." I shrug, looking down at her. Her baby blue eyes are filled with tears, and I can say for sure this time that they are happy ones. I kiss her nose, and she closes her eyes. Tears roll down her cheeks, and she wipes them away before she sniffs.

"You say the sappiest things." She smiles.

"Only to you."

"Oh, look!" she yells and points into the yard. "Lightning bugs! I used to capture them when I was a kid and put them in a jar. Go get a jar, baby, please." She jumps up from the swing. I run inside and grab two jars from the kitchen.

"Here," I say, walking out onto the porch. She is in the yard, and I stare at her as she chases fireflies in the dark. Her curls bounce, and she catches one in her hand. They light up all around her. It's the most beautiful sight I've ever seen—wild curls, pretty bugs, and a sky filled with stars.

Chapter Three
Cash

The lights have been cut on so I make Sara breakfast and take it upstairs. "Baby," I say, tapping on the door to our room. "I've brought you breakfast. Can you get up and eat?"

"I just can't today." She turns away from me. "I'm sorry. I just…can't."

"But I made you breakfast," I say. She sits up.

"Cash, don't you think I'd eat if I could? Don't you think I'd get up if I could?"

"You can."

"Please leave me alone," she says, rolling over and covering herself with the blanket. I walk in and place the food on her nightstand. I see tears on her cheeks, and I feel useless.

"I'm sorry," she cries.

"Don't be. Just sleep a little longer, and then we'll have some lemonade on the porch swing when I get back," I say it with high hopes, but I should know better. Sara's mind is making the rules for her now, and I have no say. "I love you forever," I whisper into her ear.

"Promise?"

"Promise, promise." I kiss her hair, and with a heavy heart I walk down the stairs. Doubts run through my mind as I pass by boxes that still need to be unpacked. I sigh and grab my keys. Her parents said it over and over. *Don't move her away from here. Who will watch her when she is having a hard time and you need to leave?* I pick up the house phone and call her mom. I have to see if she can come over until I get finished down at the station. Her drive is about thirty minutes and Sara will be pissed, but I can't risk it. I just pray she sleeps until Debbie gets here.

*

I pull up to the chief's office and hop out of Old Blue. It's early morning still, and I look down the street and see people opening up their shop doors. My attention turns back in front of me when I notice a short, round lady unlocking the door that reads *Chief's Office*. She gives me a smile, and as she opens the door, I hear a bell ring.

"Well, hello," she says, holding the door open for me to walk in. The smell of coffee and flowers hits my senses as I step inside.

"Good morning."

"Would you like a cup of coffee? The chief tells me I fix the best, but you know he may just be trying to butter me up. After all, I am his wife."

"Please, and I'm sure that's not the case." I wink.

She laughs, and I see lines of age around her soft blue eyes. With that and the streaks of gray in her hair, I'd say she's in her mid-fifties, just like I'd assumed the chief was. "What brings you here?"

"He is here for a job," the chief says, walking from the back of the office.

"Good morning, sir."

"Son." He nods, then turns to his wife. "Anne, how about you print out some forms for this man to sign? You and I will go for a ride around the town," he says, looking back at me.

"I'll get on that," she replies. "I'm sorry." She shakes her head. Her cheeks turn bright red, and I know I'm going to like this woman. "I didn't even introduce myself. My name's Anne Rogers." I take her hand when she reaches it out— it's small and soft. "And this is Chief Drew Rogers."

"I'm Cash. Cash Williams," I say.

"Well, Cash Williams, it's a pleasure to meet you." The bell rings and in walks a man shorter than me with a head full of curly dark hair. He looks a lot younger than my twenty-seven years, and he has a suit on so I'm assuming he is the other deputy.

"This here is Guzman," Drew says.

I stick out my hand. "Nice to meet you. I'm Cash."

"Pleasure. Name's Ben, but everybody calls me Guzman. You can call me either or."

I nod when the chief speaks. "We'll get those papers signed when we get back, Anne. Guzman, you checking in on the Kingsleys today?"

"Headed over there now," Ben replies.

"Well, grab you some coffee first. You don't wanna offend Anne here."

"No one is offending me. You boys go along now. I need to clean up this here office. I swear, you dust, and then bam, it's right back like you didn't do anything at all."

I smile as Drew lifts his hat from the coat rack, and the bell dings when he opens the door. I grab my coffee from Anne and follow him out.

"I called your father yesterday," Drew says once we get into the car. The smell of leather and carpet cleaner fills my nose, and the inside reminds me of my dad and the times I rode around with him before I got my own car. I push those thoughts aside and look over at the chief.

"Oh, yeah?" I ask, thinking he probably ran my tag when he pulled me over.

"Yeah, I ran your plate yesterday."

Bingo.

"No offense. Just had to do a background check."

"None taken," I reply, taking a sip from my coffee cup, thinking Anne was right. This is some damn good coffee.

He nods. "Your father said he hasn't spoken to you in a good while." I see him cut his eyes to me.

I clear my throat. "Last Christmas to be exact," I say, resting my cup on my knee. "My father and I didn't see eye to eye about some things." I look out the window.

"I see," he says, stopping at a red light. "Well, I don't want to get into your business. He confirmed you working for him and put in a good word for you."

"He did, did he?" I ask, a little shocked.

"You seem surprised?" Drew says.

"I guess I am. Didn't have too many nice words for me the last time we spoke, so…"

The chief nods. “Well, I don’t see any reason why I can’t hire you. So if you want the job, it’s yours.”

“I appreciate that.”

“Now, this is a small town, and in small towns you get to know people well. You get to know the troublemakers and the couples who like to fight, the drunks and the crazy teenagers who have nothing better to do but ride around on the weekends drinking and driving. We mostly let people go with a warning. Most don’t mean no harm anyway,” he says, pressing the gas and heading straight.

“That there is Berry Hunt’s barber shop. Most of the men get their beards trimmed up and hair cut there.” He points to the small shop, and I look as we ride by. “So if you want to get yours trimmed up, that’s the place to go.” I run a hand over my short beard and look when he points farther down. “Down there is Banner’s Bar. It’s where all the locals hang out. If you want to get to know people, that’ll be a good place to do it. That’s Billy’s Barbeque Pit. He cooks the best barbeque ribs you’ll ever taste. Won a few out-of-state cooking competitions, too.” He grins.

He points again. “That’s where everyone does their grocery shopping, and most of the food is farm fresh. We got a good bit of farmers in this town, and they sell their produce and meat to Sally, the lady who owns the store."

"Yeah, the wife and I went in yesterday," I tell him.

He nods. "There's a Wal-Mart a few miles from here." He points toward the direction of the main highway. "And a bigger grocery store with a shopping mall and all. We aren't totally secluded." He grins again. "But like I said, it's a small town and we like to help each other by shopping locally. We got a few clothing stores on Third Street to keep the ladies happy and a nail salon and all that. I'm sure your wife will like them just fine. Most of the other women do." He smirks as he turns onto Fourth Street. "That's where they do all their gossiping, too." I laugh. "There's a small theater and a steakhouse if you want to take your wife out."

"Let me guess, best steaks in town?" I ask with a grin.

"See, you're getting the idea." He winks. "So, anyway, it's pretty quiet around here. We mainly just make sure it stays that way."

"Understood," I say as I take another sip of my coffee. I clear my throat as the chief turns onto the road that takes us back to the office.

*

"Well, how was the ride?" Anne asks when we walk back into the office.

"Just showed him around the town a bit," Drew says.

"You didn't blink, did you?" She laughs, looking over at me. I smile back.

"I'm used to small towns. My wife and I grew up about thirty minutes from here."

"Well, good, because you know with small towns come gossip, and everybody knows everybody, and everybody knows everybody's business. Like that saying goes, 'Everybody dies famous in a small town.' And that's the damn truth," she says, moving around her desk. "But I love this place, and most of the people are good. It's hard to find good people with a world gone to shit."

"Don't go into your the-world-is-a-bad-place talk, Anne. We don't want to run the boy off already with your yapping."

Anne laughs and pats my arm. "Sorry, son. I just get a little carried away, but it's a damn shame you can't turn on the news without hearing about another school shooting or a nut job going into one of those dance places and killing a bunch of innocent people. Anyway, just grinds my gears, is all. I've got your paperwork printed out. You just take it home with you," she says, handing me a folder. “Is your wife looking for any work?” she asks. “I know Maci needs some help down at the library a few times a week. It’s part-time, but it’ll give her something to do. That is, if she wants something to do.”

“I’ll ask her,” I reply. “But she’s on disability, so she isn’t supposed to work.”

“Oh. Well, I’m sure Maci would work something out with her. Maybe pay her under the table.”

“Woman, sometimes I think you forget that I’m the chief,” Drew says to her.

“I surely don’t,” she replies, winking at me. He shakes his head.

“Well, son, I’ll have your suit and gun ready for you Monday morning. You can start then.” He moves Anne out of the way and takes a seat in front of her desk. Reaching into a drawer, he pulls out a cigar and a box of matches.

“Sounds good. Thanks again,” I say as I walk to the door. The bell rings when I open it, and I hear Anne talking.

“Don’t you smoke that thing in here. You’ll have my allergies just a fussing.”

I can't hear what he says back, but as I'm getting into my truck I hear that bell again and the smell of a cigar being lit hits my senses.

*

The screen door opens, and Debbie walks out onto the porch. I kill the engine and get out.

"Cash." She nods to me, placing her hands on her hips

"Thanks for coming, Debbie. How is she?"

"Sleeping still," she says, crossing her sweater-covered arms over her chest. It's eighty out and this woman has on a sweater. "She won't get up, and she screamed at me. Are you giving her medicine to her?"

"I don't give it to her, Debbie. She knows to take it," I answer, walking onto the porch.

"And you're not making sure she takes it every day?" she asks me.

"She's grown." I open the screen door, knowing she'll follow me.

She huffs, "You have to make sure she's taking it, Cash. I still don't know what you two were thinking. Sara's sick. She can't be left alone. She shouldn't be sleeping. If you were making sure she's taking her medication, she wouldn't be sleeping all day like this."

"It's because of the meds she is sleeping all day like this," I say to Debbie, opening the fridge and grabbing a beer.

"So, you're drinking now?" She looks at the beer in my hand.

"If you're asking if I'm about to drink this beer, then yes. If you're implying I have a drinking problem, then no," I say, twisting the cap off and tossing it into the trash. I walk past her and back onto the porch. I hate dealing with this woman. I know Debbie is concerned about her daughter, but she could cut me some slack. I sit down on the swing and look up when she comes walking out.

"Cash, why don't y'all sell this junk pile and move back home? We can take care of Sara there. We can watch her."

"No!" I say. She jumps from the sound of my voice. "Debbie." I sigh. "I'm sorry. Thank you for coming. You should be getting on your way before it gets dark." It's only a little after lunch, but I need her to leave before I lose my shit. She gets that same defeated look in her eyes I've seen many times over and her shoulders slouch.

"Fine," she says. "Call me if you need me." She walks down the steps.

"Debbie," I call after her before she gets into her car. "Thank you."

"You never have to thank me for looking after my child," she says. I nod and she gets in. I sip my beer as I watch her leave and look over at the door as it opens. Sara walks out in her pajamas and piled-up curls.

"She's gone, huh?" she asks, sitting down beside me. The swing rocks as she folds her legs under.

"She is," I confirm.

"Why did you call her?"

"You know why, baby." She doesn't say anything because she does know why. Sometimes Sara gets bad thoughts and doesn't want to live anymore. She leans down and rests her head on my lap. I kick off the porch and drink my beer. We sit in silence as the day passes by, just looking out at the old road and the wheat fields that sway from the wind.

*

"I got the job," I tell Sara as we sit on the floor in front of the couch. We've unpacked the whole house, and our coffee table is filled with things we both love. Beef jerky has made my teeth hurt, and Sara's hands are buttered up from popcorn.

"I figured you would," she says, wiping her fingers off.

"Well, aren't you going to say congratulations?" I ask. She sighs and tosses the kitchen towel onto the table.

"Is this what you want, Cash?"

My eyes look over when a soft curl falls from behind her ear.

"Yes."

"Okay. Well, then congratulations." She unfolds her legs and stands up.

"Where are you going?" I ask as she walks away from me.

"I want a shower."

"Are you mad, Sara?" I stand, too. She doesn't respond, and I watch her walk up the stairs.

"Baby," I call, following her. "Sara, I want you to be okay with this. I need you to be okay with this."

"I'm fine!" she yells and shuts the bathroom door harder than I'd like. I decide to follow some more. The sound of running water flows through my ears when I come near the door. I tap on it.

"Can we talk about this?"

"No." I hear, and as I go to twist the doorknob, the door flies open. "You know what?" she says and my eyes look down at her in nothing but boy shorts and a black bra. "I've changed my mind. We can talk about this." Mad love rushes past me, and I turn around. "You never even discussed this with me," she says, pacing back and forth. "You didn't say, 'Sara, when we move I'm going to get another cop job.' You just stuck your head right out of that stupid window and asked the chief if he was hiring. I wasn't even included in the conversation, Cash. You act as if I'm a child. I am an adult, baby. A grown woman!" she yells.

"I know that."

"Oh, you know, do you?" she replies, all smart-ass. "If you know I'm a grown woman, then why don't you treat me as one? I'm sick, Cash, not stupid."

"I've never called you stupid," I say, deadpan.

"You don't have to." She crosses her arms. I step toward her, and she steps back.

"Sara."

"Cash," she replies, turning her head sideways and lifting her brow. I step forward again, and she moves her foot back.

"Stop moving away from me."

"I don't think so, Mr. Deputy. I think I will move away from you, and I think I'll sleep away from you, too."

I know wrinkles are now on my forehead, and I narrow my eyes. "So, you're not going to sleep in the same bed as me?"

"Nope. You, my husband, will sleep on the couch down there with the mice!" she says, like *ha!*

"Oh, really?" I question with a lift of my brow line. This time she narrows her eyes when I step forward again.

"Cash," she warns and backs up two steps.

"Where are you going?" I ask her as I step forward again. I see it when her emotions betray her, and a small smile tugs at the corners of her lips. I launch forward, and she squeals as she takes off running. I chase her down the stairs and grab her just as she turns into the kitchen. "Don't ever run from me, Sara."

"Put me down."

"Nope." I smack her ass and set her down on the table. Putting my arms at her sides, I cage her in and search her pretty blues.

"I'm sorry," I say. She goes to speak, and I quickly put my finger over her lips. She clamps her mouth shut. "From now on, I won't do things without discussing them with you first."

"Can I speak now?" she mouths behind my finger.

"Yes."

"So, no more calling my mother without asking me?"

I sigh. "Sara, I do that to make sure you're safe. I couldn't bare it if you…"

"I know," she says sadly. She exhales and puts her hands on her thighs. "My water is getting cold."

"Go take your shower then." I move to the side so she can stand.

*

"I wanted to tell you earlier, but you were mad at me."

"With good reason," she says, looking over at me. We're hanging our white curtains in our bedroom. They smell like clean linens and are still damp from the wash. Sara wants them to dry while hanging so the room will smell good.

"With good reason," I repeat with an eye roll. "Anne, Chief Rogers' wife, wanted to know if you were interested in a job down at the library. I told her I'd ask you. She said you could probably get paid under the table." I chew the inside of my cheek, waiting for her to blow up. She looks back down at the curtain as she slides it onto the rod and sucks her bottom lip in.

"All right," she says after a moment. "I think it'll be good."

"Really?" I ask, shocked as hell.

"Yes, I'll give it a try."

"Okay," I say, swallowing. "I'll call Anne tomorrow."

She hands me the curtain rod, and I reach up and put it above the window.

"Now," she says, letting up the windows. "Let's let the breeze dry them."

Chapter Four
Cash

Sweat slides down my back, and my muscles burn from overuse. I wipe my brow and pick up the hammer. Another nail goes into a new board, and I sit back on my heels. I look out at my wife who is working in her new garden.

"How's it going over there?" She's in her green hat and a T-shirt that says something about coffee and don't talk to me before. A long skirt covers her legs, and I know she is barefoot because she doesn't like shoes. Her hands are covered in dirt even though she has garden gloves. She says she likes the feel of the cool soil between her fingers.

"Hot," she replies. "Want a break?"

"Yes, I'll grab us two beers. Come up on the porch." I let the screen door shut behind me, and I see Sara sitting on the step as I walk over with two cold ones in my hands.

"Didn't wanna wash your hands?" I ask as I take a seat beside her and look down at the dirt under her nails.

"Figured they were just going to get dirty again."

I smile. "You've got a point." I twist the top off and give her one before I open mine, too.

She swipes her hand in front of her face. "God dang bees."

"They're just wood bees, baby. They won't hurt you."

"I don't want them flying in my face, though."

We both look up when someone pulls into the driveway.

"Who is that?" Wood bee hater asks.

"I don't know." I stand up just as a guy gets out of his truck, and I see it's Mark from the hardware store.

"Hey there, you two."

"What brings you out this way?" I ask, walking down the steps.

"Oh, just wanted to see if I could give you a hand on this old house. I see you've been working?"

"Yep." I turn to look back at the porch. "Just replacing some old boards."

"Well, you wanting any help?"

"I couldn't put you out like that."

"You'd be doing me a favor. My wife has ten dogs at the house right now. Says she wanted to get them all bathed because they go to new homes tomorrow. Don't know why she has to do it at our house. She works at the animal shelter downtown, always bringing pets home," he says, shaking his head. I laugh and so does Sara.

"I guess if you don't mind, I'd probably get done a lot faster."

"Let me just grab my tool belt." He walks back to his truck, and I take a sip of my beer.

"Time to do man work, baby." This makes her laugh.

"Well, you get to it then."

"You down the rest of this beer for me."

"I'll do my best." She winks.

*

"What made you two want to move to a small town like Green Ridge?"

"Just needed a change, is all. We grew up about thirty minutes from here, in a small town just like this one."

"Really, and y'all wanted to move to another? Man, my wife would love to leave here and move to the city. Can't tell you how many times I've heard it."

"Sara wouldn't care for the city."

"Why is that?" he asks. I lean up on my knees and run a hand over my face, feeling I need a trim soon. Truth is, Sara gets anxiety around too many people. Large crowds make her uncomfortable, and sometimes she has panic attacks. So we decided to pick a small town on the map not extremely far from home. We picked here and packed everything up. Sara's mom almost killed me. She smothered my girl, and everyone saw it but her. But I don't know this man enough to talk about my wife's issues. Maybe one day I will.

"If you don't want to talk about it, it's fine." He reads my mind.

"Just too crowded," I say, grabbing another nail.

"That's exactly how I feel. Can't get to know people when there are too many of them."

"You said your wife works at the animal shelter?" I ask, changing the subject.

"Yeah, on Fifth Street. Been there since we graduated high school. She seems like a hard ass, but she's a softy. Like I said, brings home stray animals all the damn time. Thankfully, she's good at finding permanent homes for them or else we'd be overrun." He laughs as he nails another board in. "You know, a tin roof would look good on this house. Something to think about for the future."

"I'll keep that in mind," I say.

*

The sun starts to go down and the crickets start to chirp, so we pick up the old boards and Mark helps me load them onto the back of Old Blue to take off tomorrow.

"Come on over to the house this weekend. We'll get the grill out, and I'll buy a few steaks to pay you for the work you helped me with today."

"Only if you let me do the grilling," Mark says.

"Deal." I shake his hand, and he gets into his truck.

"See y'all Saturday," he says before he cranks it. I give him a wave goodbye and walk over to the ladder and fold it up before I head over to Sara.

"You about done over here, girl?" I ask.

"Yes, my fingers are filthy. I'll never be able to get this dirt out from under my nails."

"Should have worn gloves."

"I don't like to. You know that." She goes to stand and makes a groaning noise. "I'm getting old, baby."

"Come on, you old lady." I grab her and throw her over my shoulder. She laughs.

"Cash, you're all sweaty!"

"You like it." I smack her ass and haul her inside.

*

I draw small circles on my wife's back as we lie in bed together. We're shower clean and sleepy from a hard day's work. We had breakfast for supper, and she is almost asleep. Tomorrow, I'll take her to the library. I hope it goes well. She needs to meet new people, and she needs to have friends. I know it's scary for her, but hopefully she can overcome her anxiety. She moves and snuggles down deeper into the covers.

"You sleepy, baby?"

"Hmm," is all she can manage. I reach over, turn the lamp off, and pull her closer to me. I kiss her hair and close my eyes, letting the day finally come to an end.

Chapter Five
Cash

I park the truck and look over at Sara. "You sure you're going to be okay?" I ask, turning toward her.

"Yes, Cash, I'll be fine."

"Okay, I'll pick you up whenever you need me to."

She nods and her hand comes up to her lips. I see a small shake, but I don't mention it. Asking someone about their panic attacks seems to make it worse, so I ignore the tremble in my girl's fingers.

"I'll call you." She leans over, and I give her a kiss before she opens the truck door.

"I love you."

"Love you, too."

I watch her get out, and I don't leave until she is inside.

*

Sara

Tingles run up my spine and chase each other down my arms. They crawl up my neck and spread throughout my face, like a tiny needle pricking me. I swallow the rising panic and tell myself to breathe. *It's just a library, Sara. No one is even here.* Calming down my racing heart, I try to suck in air, but it's becoming a struggle. A cold sweat coats my back, and I feel it trickle down my skin.

"Can I help you?" I hear and turn around to find a woman in a white blouse and blue jeans. "Are you okay? You look like you're about to pass out. Here, sit down." She pulls out a chair, and I take a seat. "I'm getting you some water. Take deep breaths."

I try to do just that, focusing on one spot and willing my lungs to fill with air. She comes back with water, and I grab it from her to cool my throat. "Thank you," I manage.

"Sure." She smiles, but it's a worried smile. Her green eyes show kindness, and I get a sense of calmness as I look into them. My heartbeat slows, and my lungs work normally. The shaking in my hands stops, and I take a deep breath.

"Feel any better?"

"Yes, thank you," I say, wiping my brow.

"Good. You were having a panic attack?"

"Yes."

She nods. "I used to get those all the time over the strangest things when I was pregnant."

"They do come at the worst times." I take another sip of my water.

"One time I had one at the Dairy Queen drive-thru because I couldn't figure out what kind of ice cream I wanted." She laughs, and I smile. "My name's Maci."

Oh crap, now I'm extremely embarrassed.

"I'm Sara." I wince.

"Oh, the Sara that Anne called about?"

"Yep, panic attacks and all." I look down at the floor, waiting to crawl into a black hole.

"Please don't think any more about that," she says and I look up. She smiles. "It's nice to meet you. Come on. Let me show you around." She tucks a piece of her red hair behind her ear. "This place is old as dirt, but I think that's what gives it character. It used to be a house way back when so we actually have a full kitchen here." She points toward the back. "We host book fairs and try to encourage people to donate old books they no longer want. We also have reading time for the kids." She shows me the area with big colorful pillows. "Our restroom has a small leak in the roof, so we try to keep a bucket on the floor. Don't wanna make the floor bad, too. Mark says he's going to fix it, but life gets busy. Have you met Mark and Leigh Phillips yet?"

"I've met Mark, but not Leigh."

"Oh, Leigh is great, but watch out. She'll try to send you home with a stray animal." She laughs. "She works at the animal shelter downtown, always trying to give those babies a home."

"I've heard," I say, smiling.

"Mark must have told you."

"Yeah, he came over and helped my husband replace some old boards on our porch. Said Leigh had ten dogs at their house, and he had to get out of there."

Maci laughs. "That sounds about right. But like I said, Leigh is really great. When I was pregnant, she made me a baby blanket filled with pictures of children's books on it."

"How old is your kid?" I ask.

"I lost our baby."

"That must have been hard," I say sadly.

"It was." She looks down for a moment and then clears her throat. "So, anyway, Anne said you needed to be paid under the table?"

"Yes, but if that's an issue, I totally understand."

"No, I'm just glad to have some company around here." She smiles and links her fingers together. "Now it'll only be part-time and the pay won't be great, but it'll give you something to do. So if you want it, the job is yours."

"I do. Thank you."

"Okay, good. That's settled. Let me show you how everything works. It's very easy. I'm sure you will get it quickly."

I smile as I follow her around to the desk. Cash will be happy about this. It doesn't seem like it will be full of people often, so I think I can handle it. I'm doing this for Cash. I want to be something he can be proud of and not so much of a burden on him. He would never say it, but I know sometimes he wishes I wasn't so messed up. I wish I wasn't so messed up.

"What does your husband do?" Maci asks, taking me away from my thoughts.

"He's a deputy. Works with Chief Rogers now."

"Oh, good. We don't have much crime around here, thank God, but it's good the chief has some extra help. He's getting older, been the chief as long as I can remember."

"You grew up here?" I ask.

"Yep. I love this town, couldn't imagine living anywhere else," she says. "Now, let me show you how our computer system works."

*

"Hey." I hear and look up from the computer.

"Hey," I reply, smiling at my husband.

"Good day?" he asks as he walks closer to me.

"Better than I thought." He kisses me quickly, and I look up when Maci comes around the corner.

"Hello." She smiles. "You must be Sara's husband."

"Nice to meet you. Maci, is it?"

"Yes."

"I'm Cash." He reaches for her hand to shake.

"I heard you're working with the chief. I was telling Sara I'm glad to see Chief Rogers has some more help over there," she says, taking my husband's hand. Cash smiles. "Sara, I'll close up. You two can head on home. Enjoy your evening."

"Thank you."

"I'll see you tomorrow?" she asks.

"I'll be here."

*

"So, do you think you're going to like it?"

"I think so. It's quiet, which is a plus."

"I'm happy you're happy." He smiles at me. "What do you wanna do for supper? Wanna try Billy's Barbeque Pit? I've heard they have the best ribs."

"Okay," I reply as we pull up to our house.

"I'll get changed and we can leave," he says, walking up the stairs.

✦

Cash

I open the door and let my wife walk in first. She links our fingers, and I see it when people look our way. Sara is a beauty, but she doesn't like the attention. And because she is a beauty, that's all she gets. She goes without makeup most of the time even though that doesn't matter. She looks good with or without it.

"How many?" the hostess asks.

"Two," I tell her. I look over the crowded room. "You got anything outside?" She looks at me like I'm crazy. Although it's warm today, I want my wife to be comfortable while she eats, and I know she won't be if she thinks people are looking at her.

"Right this way."

We take our seats, and I sigh happily when I notice a small fan rotating not too far from us.

"Your waitress will be over soon."

We look over the menu, and I decide on the rib plate while Sara says she wants the same.

"Thanks for asking for a seat outside," she says.

"I thought it would be better out here."

"I know you did it for me, Cash. Thank you."

"You don't have to thank me for looking out for you, Sara."

"You know I used to be worse than this?" She looks down and tugs at my heartstrings.

"I remember," I tell her. She did used to be worse. Sara found out she had manic depression when she was only sixteen. She was outgoing and into everything. Cheerleader, played soccer, and had tons of friends. She was the life of the party, and that's how I fell in love with her.

I remember the day I fell for her. A bunch of us kids were hanging out at Lake Side, and on a dare she got on the old train bridge and jumped off into the water. Most kids wouldn't do this, as it's very high up and not exactly safe. But Sara didn't care. She was wild, full of life, and when she had her mind made up, you couldn't stop her. I thought, *wow, this girl is crazy*. Crazy beautiful, crazy fun, and I was crazy in love. She is my crazy heart.

No one had any idea that my girl had secrets, that on the inside she was like a tornado—unpredictable and all over the place. Her parents knew something was up, and I knew something was up. Why was this girl so high-strung all the time? And why sometimes couldn't she muster up the energy to get out of bed?

*

"Sara is asleep, Cash. She doesn't feel well."

"She's been sleeping all day, though." I stand at the front door in a full suit, ready to take my girl to prom, but she can't get out of bed today.

"Well, I'll tell her to call you when she wakes up." Debbie goes to shut the door, but I stop her.

"Mrs. Debbie, I don't mean to be disrespectful here, but I promised Sara a dance, and I plan on giving her that dance." I look her square in her heart-shaped face.

"Let the boy by, Debbie." I hear and see Mr. Walter walk up. "Sara needs to experience normal things."

"She does experience normal things."

"What she is doing right now isn't normal. She has been in the bed for three damn days. Let the boy by."

Debbie looks pissed, but Walter doesn't back down.

"Fine," she huffs before she takes off past me.

Walter grabs the keys. "Son, I'm taking Debbie for a long drive. You seem to make my girl smile, and she needs to smile more." He pats my shoulder as he walks out and the door shuts behind me when I step in. I take a breath as I hear Debbie fussing, but then two car doors shut. I look up at the stairs and bite my lip.

My knuckle taps on the door, but I hear nothing. I tap again and still nothing, so I walk in. It's pitch-black in here, and the only sound is the fan circulating in the corner.

"Sara," I say when I make it over to her bed. She groans, but doesn't wake. "Sara, wake up." My eyes have adjusted, and I see hers blink open.

"Cash?" she questions as she rubs her head and turns over. "What are you doing here?"

"It's prom night."

"I can't go," she tells me.

"I've brought it to you, baby."

"Cash..." She tries to argue.

"Stop. You're not missing out, and I'm not either."

She sits up and moves her wild curls out of her face.

"You're all dressed up."

"And you look pretty as ever," I say. "Come on. I want to dance with you."

She moves the covers to the side, and I take her hand to pull her up. "Where's your CD player?"

"Over there." She points. I lean down and turn the small lamp on before walking over to the radio. I put in Prince, and as the music starts, I see my girl smile.

"'Purple Rain'?"

"The best." I grin. She shakes her head, and I take her hands in mine.

"I'm sorry. I couldn't get up today."

"I'm sorry you couldn't either," I tell her. Her hands go around my neck, and I put mine on her hips. As Prince croons about not wanting to cause anyone any pain, my girl leans in closer and I feel everything—the soft sway of her hips and her PJs against my hands. Her fingers readjust against the skin on my neck, and I look down into her blue eyes as she looks at my lips. Leaning down, I kiss her and hear her inhale deeply as I pull her to me. She tastes like minty toothpaste, letting me know she did get up at one point to brush her teeth, which makes me happy. I hate thinking of her in bed all day, alone. She pulls away.

"Do you love me, Cash?"

"Yes."

"Show me," she says. I search her face, looking for any hesitation, but see none. She pulls me to the bed, and I climb on top of her. On shaky arms, I hold myself up and she smiles. I don't see it often when she is down like this, so it makes my heartbeat pick up. I smile back and lean down to taste her again. Her legs fall open, and I sink between them, gripping her thigh as she links her ankles behind my back. I try to kiss her sadness away, and with my lips I try to tell her how much I love her. She moans when I press into her. I lean back on my heels, taking my blazer off and unbuttoning my shirt. She helps me slide it over my shoulders, but I keep my undershirt on. Her hands go to my belt, and I grab my wallet out from my back pocket. I take the condom out and rip it open with my teeth. She moves up and slides the cotton down her legs. I help pull it off of her. I unzip my pants, and once the condom is on, I look back at her.

"I love you, Sara. I love everything sad and happy about you."

"Promise?"

"I promise. Hold on to me, baby."

She does, and I slowly sink inside her. Her eyes shut, and I see pain in her face. She leans up into my neck, and I press forward.

"I'm sorry," I tell her as I sink all the way in. I stay still for a moment, letting her get used to me, and when she shifts upward, I move and it's every fucking thing I thought it would be, and more.

"Cash?" I clear my throat and look up. "Where did you go, baby?"

"Prom night," I say.

She blushes, and as our food comes to the table, I think I can't get done fast enough. I want my wife now.

*

Slamming the door shut, I grab Sara and press her up against the wall. "I need you, baby."

"Have me then," she says, and that's all I hear. On a grin I lift her and take her up the stairs. Our clothes come off, our lips find each other, and as I lay her down, I sink inside and make her see fucking stars.

Chapter Six
Cash

Loud buzzing and soft clipping reverberate throughout the shop, and I lean back as Berry gets to work on my beard. "Just a trim, Berry."

"Yes, sir.'"

I look over when the door chimes open, and in walks a tall man with dirty blond hair.

"Berry." He nods toward the man working on my beard.

"Lucas," Berry returns. "How's the wife doing?"

"Maci's fine."

"Maci?" I question. "Are you Maci's husband?"

"Who wants to know?"

"I'm Cash, Sara's husband. Your wife just hired mine on at the library."

He laughs once. "Right, she's the one who had a panic attack on her first day," he says, taking a seat beside Ben who has his eyes on the newspaper. I tilt my head and narrow my eyes, feeling my neck get hot.

"Lucas, no one needs any trouble around here," Berry warns.

"Just telling the truth there, boss." Lucas holds up his hands.

Ben clears his throat. "Why don't you head on somewhere else? I'm sure the diner has some coffee waiting on you."

"Why don't you pretend like you're an actual cop and go do some cop work?"

I eyeball Lucas as I wait for Berry to finish. Ben looks back at his newspaper. A hot towel is placed onto my throat, and I give it a minute before I remove it.

"That's good, Berry. What do I owe you?"

"This one is on the house, deputy."

"Thank you," I say, standing.

"Ah, we got another Barney Fife on our hands, boys," Lucas says. I look over at him.

"Good to see ol' Chief Rogers and Guz have hired on some help. Too bad it's not someone more…" he looks me over, "qualified." He sniffs and spits into the trashcan beside him. "Guess I'll see you around, buddy." He grins. I chuckle without humor and walk toward the door. Before I open it, I turn back around.

"Lucas?"

"Yeah?"

"Speak unkindly about my wife again and I'll break your fucking nose...*buddy*." I push the door open and let it shut behind me. Ben walks out and cracks a smile.

"Haven't seen anyone stand up to that piece of shit in a long time. I heard the last man that did got his arm broke, and that was back when Lucas was in high school," he tells me.

I shake my head at Ben's excitement. "Guy seems like an asshole and a bully," I say as I walk to the truck. I know I shouldn't have let the man get to me, but I don't cope well with someone talking shit about my wife.

"Cash, toss me the ball." I glance back at Mason and bounce the ball his way. He jumps and makes the shot easily. I look over when Sara and her friends sit down on the bleachers. She's wearing baggy clothes today, and her hair probably hasn't even been brushed. It's a bad day for her, but I still give her a smile.

The ball gets bounced back to me, and I catch it. "Why do you want anything to do with that girl?" Mason asks me.

"What the hell do you mean?"

"I mean, she's weird, man. Everyone knows she sleeps for days, and then one minute she's all over the place. Hell, the teachers even talk about her. I heard Mrs. Roberts telling Mrs. Bailey the girl can't even pay attention sometimes. How she is popular I don't understand it."

My mind doesn't tell my hands to stop before I throw the ball at his face.

"Don't talk about my girl, man," I say as he holds his busted nose.

*

I pull up to the house and see the screen door open. Putting the truck in park, I step out and walk inside. "Sara?" I call out as I walk through the living room. There's no answer, and I run up the stairs. The bed is unmade, and our pillows are wrapped up in the sheets. A light breeze blows the white curtains in our bedroom, and a slow panic spreads throughout my chest. I walk over to the window and look out. The moonlight shines bright, and I see that the field is empty, but a chill runs down my spine as a bad feeling passes through my mind.

Moving away from the window, I turn around and run back down the stairs. I push the door open and step out onto the porch. Looking down the road, I take off toward my truck and jump inside. My headlights shine down the road ahead of me, and my neck hairs prickle as I wonder where my wife is. As I twist my hands around the steering wheel, a cold sweat breaks out across my forehead, and I let out a sob of relief when I see my baby walking. I yank the truck in park once I hit the brake and then jump out.

"Sara," I say as I run up to her. I grab her from behind, and my eyes look down at her bare feet. "Baby, you have no shoes on."

"I don't like shoes," she mumbles, and I let out a sad laugh.

"Let me take you home." I lift her in my arms, and she lays her head on my chest. "Fucking hell, you scared me."

"I was lonely," she whispers and everything is quiet, but the sound of my heart breaking can be heard from miles away.

*

Bubbles surround my girl as I lightly run the sponge over her back. "Feel better?" I ask.

"No, everything hurts and nothing hurts at all." She hugs her knees and rests her chin on top of her hand. Her dirty blonde curls are piled up on her head. Small ringlets fall and soak up water from her skin. My eyes look at her neck, and I squeeze water from the sponge and let it drip down her shoulders.

"I'm sorry."

"Me, too," she says, looking down at the bubbles as they disappear slowly.

"Tell me how you feel, baby. Explain it to me."

"My mind is falling in on itself. Life seems blurry. Nothing is clear." She runs her hand over her face and rests it there.

"You know that natural hope that most people have?"

"Yes, baby."

"I don't have it. I can't seem to find a reason to want to stay."

"We need to find you someone to talk to."

"No." She sighs and looks over at me. Her blue eyes have lost their light. "It'll pass."

*

Sara

It sneaks in between the blinds and spreads throughout the room. Slowly, without permission, it taunts me. You haven't slept all night, and here I am. It laughs in my face, letting me know the rest of the world is awake. It's morning and another day has begun. I throw the covers off of me and sit up. Swiping at the unruly curls on my head, I get up and yank my curtains closed, shutting out the sunshine, because today I hate it. I lie back in my bed and pull the covers up to my chin. I hear footsteps on the stairs, and I swallow because Cash is going to make me get up.

"Sara." I hear and close my eyes tight, willing him to go away. *Leave me alone. I can't do it today.*

"You have work."

"I can't." I swallow the lump in my throat and wonder why I can't control these shifty thoughts in my head.

"Come on, baby."

"Cash, I can't do it today. I'm sure Maci will be fine without me."

"You have to do it. It's only for a few hours."

"But it hurts."

"What hurts? Tell me," he says, sitting down beside me.

"Everything," I cry.

*

My eyes are tired and red rims the edges, but I suck it up and walk inside. Cash looks like I feel on the inside—sick and tired. I'm only doing this for him, because if it were just up to me, I'd lie down and never get up.

"Hey," Maci chirps, and I put on the best fake smile I can.

"Hi."

"You okay today?" she asks warily.

"Been worse," I reply and put a loose piece of hair behind my ear.

She nods, but I see the uneasiness in her eyes. "Well, we have a whole lot of books to put in the system. A big church group donated earlier this morning."

"Oh, yeah?" I ask, trying to sound interested, trying to be normal. *Just be normal today, Sara.*

*

“Well, hello there.” I hear and look up from my label gun.

“Can I help you?” I ask the man with dirty blond hair.

“Maci around? Oh, wait,” he says, a creepy smile spreading across his face. “You must be Sara?”

I narrow my eyes. “Yes, and you are?”

“I’m Maci’s husband. Where is she?”

I look back when she comes around the corner. “Lucas,” she says and I catch the apprehension in her face. She clears her throat. “Sara, this is Lucas, my husband.”

“Nice to meet you,” I say.

“And you. Hey, you seeing somebody about those panic attacks? You know, Maci had ’em real bad—”

“Lucas,” she scowls. He looks at her as though she’s lost her mind.

“Don’t interrupt me when I’m talking,” he says hatefully.

“Is there something you need?” she asks, looking embarrassed. “Can we talk in the back?” He nods as she turns around and shoots me an apologetic look. I give her a small smile and look back at him as he follows her out.

*

"Pleasure meeting you, Sara," Lucas says as he walks out of the library. I nod and look back at Maci.

"Sara, I'm so sorry for what he said earlier. I didn't tell him that so he could mock you. I simply said it in a way of remembering when I had them. I didn't know he would—"

"It's okay, Maci," I cut her off. "I know I haven't known you long, but I know you meant no harm." I look away for a moment and bite my lip. "Does he treat you like that often?" I ask, directing my eyes back to her.

"It's just Lucas. He doesn't mean anything by it. Are you finished with the labels?" she asks, brushing my question off.

"Yes." I look down at the stack of books I've completed.

"Okay." She sighs, tucking a piece of hair behind her ear. "You can call it a day if you want. There isn't much more to do here."

"Are you sure? I can stay."

"Yeah, I'm probably going to leave soon also. It's a slow day, and I feel a migraine coming on." She rubs her temple and inhales a deep breath.

"All right," I say, neatly arranging the books. "You should come to the cookout we're having."

"Okay, I just might do that."

"We are living in the old house on Eighteenth," I tell her as I head for the door.

"I'll remember. Thanks, Sara."

"Sure." I walk out and then remember I have no ride. It's earlier than I normally leave, so Cash is still at work. Maybe I can walk over to the office and see if he can give me a quick lift home. I step outside and run a hand through my hair. Squinting from the sunlight, I step out onto the sidewalk and make my way to the office. Passing by streetlamps and people who seem to have a permanent smile on their faces, I nod politely and wonder why everyone is so happy. I cross my arms as I walk and look around. I pass by a small bar and hear laughter and music flowing out of it. I keep going, making my way by a barbershop and some small boutiques. Baskets of fruit sit outside a local grocery store, and flowers hang down from the streetlamps in large flowerpots. It's like Stars Hollow from *Gilmore Girls*.

*

I open the door to the chief's office, and a little bell rings above my head.

"Hello," a short, pretty lady says.

"Hi, I'm Cash's wife. I got off early and wanted to see if he could give me a ride home."

"Oh, it's so nice to meet you! I'm Anne Rogers, Chief Rogers's wife." She sticks out her hand for me to shake, and I give her a good smile. I don't want to embarrass Cash. I look like shit, but there's nothing to be done about that.

"It's nice to meet you also."

"Here, have a seat and I'll give him a call."

"Thank you."

I take my seat across from her and look around the big enough office. I see a hallway heading toward the back, and there are flowers placed wherever she can possibly fit them. On the filing cabinet, on the coffee table, on her desk, and there's even a table just for flowers.

After she gets off the phone, she clears her throat. "Cash will be just a little bit. He's dealing with the Kingsleys. Those two can never get along. They fight until sunrise, and then they make up and sleep all day." She laughs. "Would you like some coffee? I know it's a little late for it, but it's still fresh. I make it all day for Drew."

"I would love some," I reply, still feeling the tiredness from getting no sleep last night.

"I'll fix it for you. Sugar or cream?"

"Just black, thank you. I see you're good with flowers?"

"Oh, yes, dear. I love me some flowers."

"Anything you can teach me? I'm trying to grow a small garden."

"Of course. Do you have good soil? They say success is in the soil."

"I think so."

"And what about sunlight? Flowers need a lot of energy to grow. I set mine outside on the sidewalk in the afternoons when the sun shines in front of the office." She hands me my coffee and takes a seat back in front of her desk.

"Yes. There is plenty of sunshine." I sip my coffee and hold the cup on my knee.

"Oh, good. Well, I'll tell ya one thing. Don't water those babies at midday. It'll sunburn them. Also, if you get you a little Epsom salt and sprinkle it over your soil, it'll make your plants grow healthier. Coffee grinds are good for it, too."

"Don't you be listening to Anne's old wives' tales." I hear and turn around to see the chief standing by the coffeemaker.

"How do think my flowers got so pretty, Drew?" she says.

"'Cause I buy you Miracle-Gro." He smiles and winks over at me.

"You do not!" she says sternly. He laughs and I can't help but smile a little, and it's actually genuine.

"So, what made you get off earlier today?" Anne asks me.

"Maci said she was getting a migraine and wanted to close up early." I shrug.

"Oh," she says, and I see her give Drew a look. I don't question it, though. The bell on the door rings, and I see my husband.

"Hey." He smiles, and his smile is always authentic when he looks at me.

"Hey, baby," I reply.

"Cash, your wife and I were just talking about growing a garden. She says she has one started at your place."

"Yes, ma'am, she does."

"How'd it go at the Kingsley's place?" Drew asks me.

"Fine. They had a little too much liquor, and Joe broke the coffee table when he fell on it. He tripped over Elizabeth's shoe, and that pissed him off, so he started yelling at her. She started crying and throwing old bread at him, which made him madder because it had mold on it. The neighbors got tired of the screaming, so that's why they called."

I laugh. "She threw moldy bread at him?" Cash grins at me.

"Yep, you ready to go?"

"Yes. Anne, thank you for the coffee. It was the best I've had."

"Oh, I'm happy you liked it." She beams and takes the empty cup from me. "I hope to see you again. Let me know if I need to come get my hands dirty."

"Yes, ma'am."

*

"Remember when you were seventeen and got busted for climbing the water tower?"

"Yes," I say, remembering back to what seems like a lifetime ago. "First time I was ever in a cop car."

"But not the last," Cash says as we head toward our place.

"No, not the last." I roll down my window and let the summer breeze blow through my wild curls. As I look out at all the farmland, my mind drifts back to too many Solo cups and a reckless night.

*

"I'm not going to get caught," I tell Cash.

"Baby, I don't care about you getting caught. Well, I do, but I care more about you getting hurt."

"Oh, don't be such a worrywart. You sound like my mama," I throw back at him as I take the last sip of my beer and toss my cup to the side. My hands touch cold iron, and I grip onto the bars as I lift my feet off the ground. I shift my hands and grab onto another bar. Lifting my feet again, I begin to climb the tall tower. I look back down as Cash gets smaller and smaller, and soon he is so small I can't even see the redness in his eyes from too many beers. My hair moves off of my shoulder as a cooler than normal summertime wind moves through it and brushes it across my face. I inhale deeply and keep

going. I feel the sway of the tower the higher I get, and I can't help but think this is freedom.

There's something about being in control of your own life. I'm never in control of my mind, but at this moment I hold the power. If I release the bars, I probably wouldn't even feel the impact. I make it to the top and step onto the platform. Spreading my arms wide, I close my eyes, and a strong urge passes through me to let go, jump. It'll feel like flying, *my mind says, but falling only feels like flying until you hit the ground. I look down when I see blue lights.*

"Oh shit, Mama is going to be pissed."

Chapter Seven
Cash

I stretch my arm across the bed, feeling for Sara. My eyes shoot open when I realize she isn't here, and like always my heart picks up beats. I sit up, running a hand over my face, and toss the covers off. I look toward the bathroom and see the light isn't on behind the closed door. She isn't there either.

"Sara," I call out, but no response. I get up, and when I open the door, I hear music. As I make my way downstairs, light blinds me and I have to shield my eyes. Almost every light in the house is on. "Sara?" Still no answer. I continue down the steps and round the corner. Sara is on her hands and knees scrubbing the kitchen floor. Wearing old sweats and a T-shirt that's tied up on the side, she sings along to the music, and I see sweat running down her face. "Sara, what the hell are you doing?" She still doesn't hear me and obviously doesn't realize I'm up. I walk over and stop the record player. She falls back.

"Shit, Cash." Her hand comes to her heart, and she sits on her butt. "You scared the piss out of me." She tosses her dirty towel into the bucket, and I move out of the way as water splashes onto the floor. "I'm sorry. Was the music too loud?"

"What are you doing? It's four in the morning."

She puffs a fallen piece of hair out of her face. "This floor is super dirty," she says, waving her hand at it. "And so is the rest of the house… well, was…" She looks over the hardwood and shrugs.

"So, you clean it now?" I look at her like she has lost it, and maybe this time she has.

"I can't freaking sleep. I tossed and turned for two hours, and then I remembered how I wanted to clean the floors, and then I said I might as well clean the cabinets, too."

I look up and see all the plates and glasses sitting out on the counter.

"Sara, this is crazy. You're going to feel like shit later today."

"No, I'm good. I'm really good," she says, grabbing her towel back out of her bucket and wringing it out. She gets back on her knees and continues scrubbing.

"But you haven't slept."

"I'm telling you, Cash. I feel great. I'm just going to get the house ready for later. We won't have to clean a thing." I stare down at her as she wrings out her towel again and does a wax on, wax off motion.

"Have you been taking your medication?"

She looks up at me. "I don't need it."

"What the hell do you mean, you don't need it?"

"I mean, I don't freaking need it. Now, get out of the way. You're tracking. Did you wash your feet tonight?"

"This is not good."

She sighs and rolls her eyes, sitting back on her heels. "If I was feeling like shit, wouldn't I tell you? Why when I feel on top of the world, do you want to bring me down?"

"I'm not trying to bring you down, baby. But this is not normal behavior. People don't get out of bed in the middle of the night and start scrubbing floors," I say, looking up at the countertops. "Or clean out cabinets."

"Why don't you go back to sleep?" She stands and walks toward me. "I'll be up in a little bit." She kisses my lips, and I look down at her. I tuck a stray piece of hair behind her ear and put my hand on her hip.

"You can't stop taking your medicine," I say softly.

"I'll start back tomorrow. Happy?"

"Yes, but I won't be happy if you keep this up all night, so I guess I'll have to help you finish."

*

The cabinets have been refilled, and the house smells like lemons and Pine Sol. Sara dances around the kitchen, smiling and talking my head off. The knees of her sweats are wet and her tied-off shirt rides up, showing a small bit of her soft skin. She gives me a look when our song comes on—a song we danced to on prom night when couldn't seem to get out of bed. I love when she has her hair pulled up in a careless way and ringlets hang down in the back and front.

"Do you remember our senior year when we skipped school and drove down to Lake Side? There wasn't a person on the lake. It was just us two."

"How could I forget? You talked me into skinny-dipping."

She laughs. "You were so nervous."

I walk over to her and wrap my arms around her waist. "You've always pulled me out of my comfort zone."

"I'm crazy," she says, turning around in my arms and looking up at me.

"Crazy beautiful," I reply before I kiss her lips. Her arms wrap around my neck, and I lift her up onto the countertop. Love runs her hands down my arms, and I try to kiss her crazy away. Her lips are soft, and her curls tickle my face. Her smell—clean and raspberries mixed—surrounds me and I breathe in, trying to make my mind engrave it so whenever I need its comfort, it'll be there. I pull her closer, and she wraps her legs around my back. Her hands go to my shirt, and I move away so she can take it off. Rosy red fingernails scratch my skin, and I grab her tied-up T-shirt and undo it. It falls loose, and I lean down and kiss her neck.

"Lift your arms." She does and I pull her cotton shirt over her head. My face goes back to her neck, and I kiss every inch of her skin I can get my lips on.

Moving her from the counter, I bring us to the floor, and she slides her sweats and panties off. Skin I love gets covered in kisses by me, and I sink two fingers inside her. The vibration of her moans is felt through my face as I lick down her chest and across her stomach. Her hands run through my hair, and she wiggles beneath me as I move my face down farther. I let my tongue explore until she can't take it anymore, and then I grab myself and lean up to kiss her mouth as I bury myself inside her. Her head falls back, and I grasp her thighs as she links her ankles behind my back. I love her crazy away, and in this moment, her mind belongs to me.

*

Charcoal burns on the grill as Mark flips the steaks over and I hand him a beer. The sun shines bright outside, but I can see a storm behind my girl's eyes. She slept for maybe two hours earlier, and you can see no rest on her face. Leigh talks with her, but as nice as Leigh seems, Sara looks uninterested, and she keeps messing with her fingers. I take a sip of my beer as the chief and Anne pull up. My wife looks over at me, and I give her a smile. It asks her if she is okay, begging her to be.

"Drew," I say as he walks up to me.

"Son." He nods and shakes mine and Mark's hands. Anne walks over to Leigh and Sara and hands my wife a bowl of something. "Anne made some potato salad. It's good. I snuck a bit before we drove over," Drew says. Mark laughs and I pretend to listen, but my attention is somewhere else. I watch Sara walk inside, and I tell the boys I'll be back. The screen door shuts behind me, and I see Sara leaning against the countertop, fingernail between her teeth. I play it cool.

"Mark's steaks are looking good," I say, walking over to the fridge. She doesn't respond.

"Want a beer?"

"No," she answers.

I nod and grab the boys and me one. "Leigh seems nice."

"Yeah."

"Is Maci coming?"

"I don't know."

"Wanna give her a call and see?"

"No, Cash. Stop asking twenty questions." She walks away from me, and I take a deep breath.

"Shit."

*

Sara sits on the porch swing while Anne and Leigh lay the tablecloth down. The steaks are done, and we are ready to eat. I take a sip of my beer and walk up the steps.

"You hungry, baby?"

"Not really," she says.

"Wanna try to eat something anyway?" I ask.

"Yeah, I'll come down." She's being antisocial, but it could be worse. At least she is out here.

*

"You did a damn good job on those steaks," I tell Mark as we clean up.

"Anytime you need a cook, just call me." He grins.

"He does most of the cooking at our house," Leigh says. "And I happily let him." She smiles at her husband and then looks over at Sara. "Honey, if you ever wanna get out of the house, you just give me a call. We can plan something."

"I'll keep that in mind. Thank you." She's quiet and drawn-in, but she compliments Anne's potato salad and tells everyone thank you for coming before she lies about having a headache and heads inside. I get looks, but I finish the cleaning.

"Your wife okay?" Mark asks.

"Yeah, she just gets headaches sometimes."

"I used to get those things," Anne says. "Ruin a whole day, they will. Keep you shut up inside a dark room. Warm baths used to help me. Maybe you should run her one, Cash. We can finish up here."

"I will in a little bit."

*

After everyone leaves, I walk up the steps and into the bedroom, thinking Sara will be lying down, but she isn't. I hear water running, and I walk into the bathroom.

"Sara!" I yell as I run over and pull her out of the water. "Fucking hell, baby." I stand her on her feet and grab a towel. She's out of it, and I see her hands shaking. I kiss her forehead and wrap the towel around her, pulling her close to me. "Sara, what were you doing?"

"I was trying to cut out the noise. It's so loud in my head," she says as she starts crying.

"Let's get out of these wet clothes and we can lie down together for a bit."

She agrees and I help her undress. She shakes and I'm not sure it's from being cold or she's just scared.

I pull a nightgown down over her head and move the covers back so she can get under. I lie down beside her and wrap my arms around her back.

"I love you, baby."

"Promise?" she asks quietly.

"Promise, promise," I whisper as I kiss her hair and pray to God she never leaves me on purpose.

*

Sara

Darkness. Black everywhere inside and out. The hardwood floor presses against my bare knees, and I stare at nothing. My mind races with scary thoughts, and I can't seem to pinpoint on just one. I lean over and tears I didn't even know were in my eyes fall out and hit the floor. I look up and wipe my face, rocking back and forth and wondering why I even bother to breathe. It hurts. "It hurts," I whisper to the darkness.

*

A week has flown by, and I've seen nothing but these walls. I'm tired all the time, yet I can't sleep, so I sit on the front porch and watch the fireflies at night. Cash constantly watches me. I want to scream at him to stop. Stop watching me. Stop looking at me. Stop beating, you stupid heart.

*

I think about dying a lot because I'm tired of hurting. I'm tired of being tired, but not sleeping.

I'm tired of my racing thoughts, and I'm tired of watching fireflies. I grab the knife and put it up against my wrist. Pressing down, I watch as red spills over my pale skin. I fall to my knees and close my eyes and wait for it to be over.

"Baby! Oh God, Baby, baby." I hear my heart speaking, but I can't feel its beats. My eyes won't open, and blackness finally takes me over. I smile on the inside because the pain will finally be over.

*

I roll over and slowly open my eyes. They find Cash, and I sigh lightly and rest my face against the palm of my hand. Seeing the bandages around my wrist, a sickness sinks inside my chest and I look away. The sun shines through the window and makes his dark hair look golden brown. I look at the wedding ring on his finger and then look for mine. It rests where it should, and I twirl it around as the nurse walks in.

"You're awake," she whispers, seeing that Cash is fast asleep.

I smile, feeling better than I have in a long time. "We have balanced out your medications and set you up with a psychiatrist, but the doctor will be in to tell you all of that. I'll let you rest and see you later on."

“Thanks,” I say before she walks out. I turn back around and see my husband’s brown eyes looking at me.

“Hey,” he says softly.

“Hey,” I reply.

“How are you feeling?”

“Just a little tired,” I say as he stands up and stretches.

“Move over. I’m getting in with you.”

I smile and move over as far as I can. He lies down, and I rest my head on his chest, hearing the beat of his heart.

“I love you and I’m sorry,” I tell him.

“Please don’t leave me,” he says.

“I won’t do it again.”

“Promise?” he asks.

“Promise, promise.”

Chapter Eight

Six Year Anniversary

Sara

This year flew by with changes of medication and tons of therapy visits. Most days I feel somewhat normal or more balanced out I should say, because really what is normal? Like all small towns, word got around about my suicide attempt, but the looks have stopped and most people have been very supportive. My wrist has healed, but the scar remains. It's deep and ugly, reminding my husband and me that I almost left him. My therapist, Dannie, suggested I keep a journal and write my feelings down every day, so I try to do that. Unfortunately, my medication makes me sleepy and also less creative in life, but we can't always get what we want. Maci totally understood and let me come back to work as soon as I was ready.

I look over as a pile of books get knocked down. "Shit." I hear Maci curse.

"Everything okay over there?"

"Yeah, just stacked them too high," she calls out. I walk over and see books surrounding the girl I now call my friend. Red hair falls into her face, and her green eyes look up at me. I laugh.

“Let me help you,” I offer. She picks up the fallen books, and I see a bruise on her arm. “Get that just now?”

She looks down at her arm and then back at the books in her hand. “I bruise so easily I have no idea where it came from.” I’d believe this except she always has bruises, and Lucas is a complete ass to her.

“Yeah, I bruise easily, too, but you always seem to have those.”

She looks up at me again and shrugs. “I’m careless.”

“And I don’t have manic depression,” I throw back at her. She sighs.

“You trying to get at something here?”

“Just worried, is all. If I was showing signs of being on a high, wouldn’t you call me out?”

“Yes.”

“Okay then.”

“So, what’s your point?”

“My point is, that son of a bitch better not be putting his hands on you.” Maci blinks at me, and I instantly feel bad. “Look, I’m sorry. I just don’t like the way he talks to you, and it worries me. I know he is your husband—”

"That's right. He is my husband and the man I love. Please don't talk about him again."

I bite my lip and look down. "I'm sorry. I won't say another word about it." I pick up the rest of the books and walk back over to the desk.

*

The summertime sun is high in the sky today, and I lie back on my float and lightly strum my fingertips over the pool water. A horsefly flies by, and I look up at the small amount of clouds.

"Have you read that book I was telling you about yet?" Leigh asks me as we float mindlessly and soak up some rays.

"I finished it last night. It was good."

"It was," she agrees as she grabs ahold of the end of my float so we stay connected. I look over at her.

"Do you think Lucas is beating Maci?" I ask. I haven't spoken to anyone about this, not even Cash because I don't want to put it out there. But I'm getting concerned for my friend, and I'm starting to wonder if he is the reason they lost their child.

"Sometimes that thought crosses my mind. Why do you ask, though?"

“It crosses mine, too.” I block the sun from my eyes. “I’ve implied it to her, and she got super defensive. Which I understand—that’s her husband, but I just think something more is going on there. He treats her like shit.”

“Well, no one can do anything unless she wants it done,” Leigh says, shaking her head. “It’s best to just not mention it unless she does.”

I sigh and rest my head back. “Guess I won’t again.”

*

I pull the string on my bikini top and let it fall to the floor. Looking at myself in the mirror, I see I got some sun today and now have a tan line. Cash walks in behind me and lifts his brow. “Got a severe tan line there.”

“That I do.” I turn the water on and wait for it to warm.

“How was your day?”

“Good,” he says, walking over to me. He kisses my mouth, and I smell beer.

“You and the boys go by Banner’s?”

“How’d you guess?”

"You smell like beer." He kisses my neck, and I feel his fingers skim across my lower back. "Want to have a quickie?"

"Yes," I breathe as his hand ventures low, and he removes my bottoms. He lightly runs his hand over me, and I lean back against the wall.

"I love you," he murmurs as he takes my lips again. His tongue dances with mine, and a moan creeps up from my chest. I hear his pants go, and in another move he has my thigh lifted and he is inside me. I grip onto his shoulders as he presses forward. Steam takes over the bathroom, and sweat drips down my back.

"God, baby," he breathes. "I fucking love the way you feel." He clutches my leg and I pull him closer, pressing my ankle into his backside. As he goes deeper, I close my eyes. I'm awed by the love he gives me, and each time he shows me, my heart beats stronger, my mind gets clearer, and my soul begs to become one with his. I love this man more than my lungs love air, and as he comes undone, I tell him over and over.

"Happy anniversary," he murmurs over my lips.

"Happy anniversary."

*

A bandana covers my eyes, and I'm directed out of the house. "Now, don't freak out on me," Cash says.

"Well, now I am," I counter. "What in the world have you done?"

"It's an anniversary gift, for both of us," he says. "Stand right here."

I inhale and get anxious as I wait for him to let me see.

"Cash," I say impatiently.

"One second," he says, standing me where he wants me before he lets my arms loose and I'm left alone. I listen as I hear his footsteps going down the porch.

"Okay, look."

Reaching up, I pull the bandana off, and my eyes find him. They grow big, and I step forward. "What in the hell is this?" I ask, smiling.

"I bought us a motorcycle, baby."

"You bought this thing?"

"Yep, so we can go riding on our days off." I walk down the steps and over to him. "It's got some age on it, but I got it at a good price, and I've had it looked at and tuned up. It's good to go." He grabs two helmets from the back. "Let's take her for a ride." He places the helmet on my head and kisses my lips. I grin like a kid who just got out of school for the summer before I hop on the back. The engine vibrates under me, and Cash tells me to hold on. I wrap my arms around his waist as he puts her in first. We circle around, and he shifts gears as we head down the old country road that needs to be repaved. My fingertips hardly touch each other, but I hold on tight as the wind tosses my hair. I smile as a feeling of freedom washes over me and I get brave. I release my hold from Cash and spread my arms out wide. Cool evening air brushes over my skin, and I close my eyes and lean my head back slightly, feeling the warmness against my face from the sunshine, thinking this is what flying must feel like. I hold on again as he goes faster and we head toward no certain destination, but after all, this is simply about the ride.

*

"I want to learn how to drive it," I say after our showers. We're lying on the living room rug with popcorn and candy.

"Okay, I'll teach you."

"Teach me now," I say, jumping up.

"It's dark out."

"So?"

"So it's dangerous. I'll teach you this weekend."

"Cash, I really wanna do it now."

"Sara," he warns.

"This isn't some stupid trigger. I just want to learn how to drive the fucking motorcycle," I say, rolling my eyes at him. He narrows his.

"You're being impatient. You're snapping on me, and you think this isn't a trigger?"

"Fuck you," I say, standing up and walking away. I climb the stairs two at a time and slam the door shut behind me. Everything is a fucking trigger to him. Can't I simply be in a bad mood? Can't I be upset without it having to do with my disorder? I grab the basket of unfolded clothes and dump them onto the bed. I sigh as my mind tells me what is true. *You can't just be upset. You're not normal. Your mood swings are extreme, and you do have triggers.* I toss the clothes to the side and sit down on the bed. The door opens, and I look up. "I'm sorry."

"Me, too," he says, taking a seat beside me. "I shouldn't think every one of your moods is more than just a mood."

"No, you should. It is what it is," I say, moving my hair out of my face.

"You will learn to drive the bike. I promise." He grabs my hand and links our fingers. I look over at him and laugh.

"What?"

"You've got popcorn in your beard."

"Get it."

I reach up and pick it out. He eats it from my hand.

"Eww."

"Why is that eww?" he asks, chewing on the popcorn.

"'Cause it's beard popcorn."

"Beard popcorn is the best, woman. Don't you know?" He grins.

"No, I don't."

"Here, let me show you."

"No," I say, trying to loosen his hold on my hand.

"Where are you going?"

"Away from your beard."

He holds my hand tighter, and I fall back as he climbs on top of me, bringing his beard down to my face and rubbing it all over me.

"You're scratching up my face." I giggle as he starts to tickle me. Placing my palm onto the bed, I try to move up and out from under him. I twist in his arms, but this only makes him do it more and hold me tighter. "Cash," I say as he tortures my sore hips. "Stop." I laugh uncontrollably and wiggle more. He quickly plants his mouth on mine, and I smile underneath his lips. My legs fall open, and he settles. I feel him grow hard beneath me, and I moan when he presses forward. "Make me feel good," I tell him, and he lifts my dress and all play leaves the room as he thrusts into me. I claw at his back, and he grabs onto the headboard, fucking me until I cry out and he goes still. Our unfolded clothes lie under us, wrinkled to hell and back, and I look over at him. He is the most beautiful thing. He is mine, and sometimes I can't believe it.

Chapter Nine
Cash

"Now, Mrs. Kingsley, you can't keep throwing stuff at Mr. Kingsley. One of these days you're going to hurt him."

"Cash, stop calling me Mrs. Kingsley. I've done told you my name is Elizabeth. And I don't throw anything at the dummy that would hurt him. Joe's just a big ol' baby," she huffs and puts her hands on her hips.

"Oh, I'm a big baby," Joe says. "What about you yesterday when you didn't get to watch your soaps because the cable went out?"

"The damn cable went out because you didn't pay it!"

"You get a job then and pay the shit. I don't even watch it!"

"You are the one who told me not to get a job, you God dang donkey!" She picks up a pillow from the couch and goes to smack him in the face, but I stop her.

"Mrs.—"

"Cash, if you call me Mrs. one more time, I'm going to hit you with this pillow."

I hold up my hands. "I'm sorry, Elizabeth. Please, put the pillow down. Now, you two love each other. You have to stop this fighting. Maybe if you stopped drinking that would help."

"We don't have a drinking problem," they both say at the same time, which tells me that's exactly what they have.

"Right," I counter, looking at empty bottles. "Do I need to take one of you in so you can cool off?"

"No," they both say.

"Well, I need you to make up then right here, right now."

"We can't do that with you watching!" Elizabeth says.

"I mean, say you're damn sorry, so I can get on my way."

"Oh, right." She blushes, and Joe smiles at her.

"You're always cute when you blush."

This makes her blush more. I step toward the door, and she puts the pillow down.

"I'm sorry for calling you a dummy," she says.

"I'm sorry for getting the cable cut off."

I don't hear the rest as I shut the door and head back to my truck. I look over at Ben when I get in. He spits a sunflower seed out the window.

"How'd it go?" he then asks me as he pours more seeds into his mouth.

"I'm sure we'll be called back over here in a few days," I answer. He smirks, and I start the truck.

*

A green hat comes into view as I pull up to our house. It's late afternoon, and the sun is low, but my sunshine is watering her sad flowers. I park the truck and jump out.

"Hey, baby," she says, tossing the water hose to the side. She runs over to me, and I catch her when she jumps into my arms. She kisses my mouth, and I breathe her in—warm sunshine and water hose water. She lets go of my lips and smiles down at me. "How was your day?"

"Better now," I tell her. She laughs, and I walk us over to the waterspout, shut the water off, and climb the steps with her still in my arms. She takes her hat off and throws it onto the couch as we pass it.

“Where are you taking me?”

“Away,” I say.

“Away?” she questions on a laugh.

“Yes, under the covers and deep inside our bed.”

She smiles. “As long as I’m surrounded by you, I don’t care.”

*

Sara walks out of the bathroom in a pale green dress and wedges. “How does this look?”

“You look good.”

She has on makeup, and her eyes shine bright. She looks beautiful, and I kiss her cherry-colored lips.

“Let’s go dancing,” she says.

*

Music from the band plays from the stage, and Sara grabs my hand and twirls around me. She joins our fingers and laughs as she dances. Her curls are wild, and her smile is infectious. I grab her close to me, and she puts her hands on my face, kissing me like no one is here, like we are the only ones on Earth. Her hands move to my hair, and she slowly runs over it, smiling at me like I'm the only thing that matters. I feel it in my chest, and I love the light in her eyes.

"Want a drink?" I ask.

"Yes," she says. We make our way over to the bar, and Banner walks up to us with a towel over his shoulder.

"Hello, you two."

"Bartender, give my husband and me two beers on tap, please, sir."

"Yes, ma'am."

"Oh, and can you put some salt on my rim?" she asks so sweetly, and I grin.

"Only for you, Sara."

"Thanks, Banner," I say as I turn toward my wife. She sways her hips to the music and moves her head side to side in the most carefree way. Nothing is bothering her today, and I send a prayer up to whomever that my girl is happy. It's written all over her face.

*

The night is long, and the girl who hates wearing shoes is barefoot as we walk down the sidewalk. She laughs at my jokes and holds my hand while her other grips her wedges. She's drunk and giddy. I'm in love and happy.

"I wish my flowers looked like these," she says, pointing to the flowers in the park. Her flowers aren't doing well, but she tries.

"Maybe Anne can come over and help?"

"Maybe so," she says, shrugging.

*

We make it home, and I carry my sleeping baby to our bedroom. I lay her in bed and then walk downstairs. Grabbing a beer out of the fridge and twisting the cap off, I head out onto the porch swing. A small breeze moves in from the field, and the old swing softly creaks as I push off with my boots. Crickets sound in the distance, and a night owl hoots from a nearby tree. I sip my beer and rest my arm against the back of the swing. The moonlight shines down on the garden Sara is trying to grow, and I get an idea. Tomorrow, I'm going to make sure my girl has some flowers.

*

I stretch my arms and roll over. Sara is still asleep, and I look and see it's early. My idea crosses my mind, and I quietly slip out of bed.

I leave a note for Sara and head out to the truck. Jumping in, I start Old Blue and make my way into town. He backfires, and I swear I'm going to get that looked at. I walk into the hardware store and make my way to the back where the flowers are.

"Hey, Cash." I look up when I see Mark standing there.

"Hey, man."

"Flower shopping?" he questions.

"Yeah, Sara isn't having any luck with her garden, so I figured I'd plant her one already grown."

He laughs. "Well, you've come to the right place. You've got a ton of sun out there, so you need flowers that can't get enough. Come on over here and we will load you up."

*

I wipe my brow and sit back on my heels. My back is sore from being bent over for an hour and a half, but I've got my girl's flowers planted, and it looks beautiful. I can't wait to see her face. She's still sleeping, so I clean up my mess and head inside for a shower. I toss the empty flower containers into the bed of the truck and slip my gloves off.

SMACK!

I look toward the house. What the hell was that?

SMACK!

I run up onto the porch and grab the handle of the screen door. I cover my mouth to hold back a laugh when I see Sara on top of a chair smacking the fly swatter up against the wall for the third time. She huffs and blows a piece of hair out of her face. The fly swarms around her before he lands back on the wall. The tips of her toes are over the edge of the chair, and she leans over as far as she possibly can. Her tongue darts out, and she draws back before she goes to smack the fly again. I run over just as she falls forward and catch her in my arms.

"Oh shit." She laughs loud, and I look down at her smiling face.

"Thank you, Cash. I'm so sick of these damn flies. I killed two, but that third one wasn't giving in."

"Glad I was here. You would have broken your face."

"Possibly," she says, quickly pressing her lips to mine. "You smell like outside."

"I've got a surprise for you."

"Another one?" She smiles as I put her down.

"Yes."

"Well, let's see it then." She puts the bug killer down, and I take her hand and walk out onto the porch. "We need to replace that screen door. There's a hole in it. That's how the bugs are getting in."

"I'll get on that."

"Also, upstairs I noticed a light was out in the bathroom… Oh, Cash." She puts her free hand over her mouth and looks from her new garden to me. "Baby, what did you do?" She lets go of my hand, and her long skirt drags the ground. I watch her face as it lights up with wonder. She turns to me. "You did all of this today?"

"Yes." I slide my hands into my pockets and bite my lip.

"It's beautiful. I've never seen anything so pretty." I watch her—the light in her eyes, the sun shining through her soft curls, the golden tan she has from lying out with Leigh. Her lips are in a permanent smile.

"I have," I tell her. She looks over my face and shakes her head.

"You amaze me."

"I never want to stop doing that."

"So don't," she says, and I walk closer to her. I take her face in my hands and kiss her lips.

"I won't," I say before I lay her down and show her just how amazing she can be.

*

"Baby, remind me to call in my meds tomorrow," Sara yells to me from downstairs.

"Will do," I call back as I remove the baked chicken from the oven. Like Mark, I'm the cook around here. Sara can burn a waffle in the toaster. She walks downstairs and grins.

"This looks so good. Can I help with anything?"

"Yeah, grab some plates, two beers, and follow me." I hear her footsteps when I push the door open, and I set the food down on the outdoor table. Lights are hung above us, and the old record player I bought plays Johnny Cash and June Carter's "Jackson".

"I love this song," Sara says after she places the plates down. She dances and laughs. I cut some chicken and place it onto our plates.

"It's a good one."

"June loved John like I love you." She takes her seat and puts her feet on my lap.

"John loved June like I love you," I tell her.

We eat in silence, just enjoying the light breeze and clear night sky. She sighs as she pushes her plate away.

"That was so good, baby."

"I'm glad you liked it. Now, you'll have to clean the dishes." I smile.

"Gladly," she says, picking up the plates and walking into the house. I watch her before I grab the other dishes and follow. Elvis plays now, and she turns around and blows soap bubbles my way as his rough voice sings about hound dogs. She laughs when some bubbles get on my nose and I shake my head.

"Stop," I tell her as she blows more.

"Stop?" she questions, throwing more at me.

"Sara, quit. You're getting bubbles all over the floor."

She grabs the sprayer and turns toward me.

"Don't you even think about it."

"Did you have a bath today, baby?" she asks, trying to hold in her laugh.

"Sara," I warn, slowly backing up.

She presses down, and water sprays my whole face. I blink my eyes open, and she squeals and drops the sprayer. She takes off running and heads toward the stairs. I run over and shut the water off before I chase her.

"You're totally getting soaked," I yell as I run up the steps. I hear the door shut, and I burst into our bedroom. She's on the other side of the bed, and I wipe a hand down my face, removing the water and rubbing droplets away from my hair.

"Cash, I was just playing now. Don't do anything crazy." She grins as I walk closer to her.

"You have nowhere to go, baby. Might as well give in now."

"Now, you know better than that."

She's all smiles and hands on her hips. She bites her lip and looks from me to the bed. I walk even closer, and she screams before she jumps onto the mattresses. I grab her leg, though, and drag her back to me. She wiggles with everything she has, but I'm stronger. I lift her over my shoulder and take her to the bathroom. She playfully slaps my back as I lean down and turn the water on. The showerhead comes on, and I step inside with her.

"Cash, that's freezing!" she screams. I slide her down my body, looking at her hard nipples through her white cotton shirt.

"No bra?" I ask.

"Well, it's just you and I." She looks up at me with those kiss-me eyes, and I look down at her lips before looking back at her blues. "You got me all wet."

"I'm about to get you wetter," I say as I slam my lips to hers. She falls back, but I catch her. Our tongues glide against each other's, and I slide her skirt down from her hips. I unbutton my soaked jeans and step out of them. She laughs when I almost fall and grabs for my arm. I kick them away and lift her, pressing her back against the tile wall. She moans when I fill her, and her head falls back. I kiss her neck and take her earlobe into my mouth, moving fast and loving the way she sounds when I do it harder. She wraps her arms around my neck, and I pound into her over and over.

"Cash, oh God." I sink us to the floor with her on top and I let her take over.

"Do you love me, Sara?" I ask.

"Yes," she breathes heavy as I lift up, rocking into her.

"Then show me," I say, throwing her words back at her from our first time. She smiles, and her hands go to her breasts as she moves, and I think I'm the luckiest son of a bitch that ever lived.

*

She lies on baby blue cotton sheets as I softly run my fingers over her skin. The curtains sway from the wind coming off the field, and I hear thunder.

"I hope this rain doesn't flood my new garden."

"I hope it doesn't either. I've already got blisters." I lift up my hand and show her. She looks over at me.

"My poor baby," she says playfully, and I roll my eyes and take my hand back.

"No, let me kiss them better," she insists.

"Nope, you lost your chance."

"Cash," she pouts, and the thunder roars again. She reaches for my hand, and I let her have it. Her lips touch my skin, and I smile over at her.

The lights blink, and Sara moves closer. “Where are the candles?” she asks.

“On the dresser. But we don’t need them.”

“Why? The lights may go out.”

“But we’re in the bed.”

“True. What if I need to go to the bathroom, though?”

“I’ve got a flashlight in my nightstand. You can put it on your side.”

“You’re going to let me have your flashlight?” she says, grinning.

“I’d let you have anything you want if it was always up to me.” I grab her naked behind and pull her on top of me.

“Will you ever get tired of me?” she asks, moving her curls out of her face. I harden beneath her, and when I move she sucks in air.

“Never,” I tell her as I move again just to hear her moan.

“Promise?” she breathes.

“Promise, promise,” I say as the rain starts to fall outside, and I love her all over.

Chapter Ten
Cash

The wind blows, and I look over at Sara as she rests her eyes. We are lying in the big field on a blanket, and the sun shines down on us. It's not hot, though. It's perfect today, and my eyes look at the scar on her wrist. I lightly grab her hand, and she opens her eyes. I press my lips to her scar, and she bunches her brow.

"Please don't ever do this again," I ask her, staring at her blue eyes.

"I'll try not to."

"I need you to swear it."

"I swear."

I search her face to see if she believes the lie she just told me. Even I know that's something she can't promise. Sometimes people lose the battle of depression. I just pray it won't be us. I don't know how I'll survive myself. I drop her hand, and she moves closer to me, wrapping her arm around my stomach. I roll over, and she lays her head on my chest. I lift my hand and lightly run it through her curls, glancing up at the vast, light blue sky. I hear a car and look out to the road. It looks like Debbie's, and I curse under my breath. "Looks like we have company," I say to my wife. She turns her head and sighs.

"What is she doing here?"

"I don't know," I reply as I stand up. "Come on."

"Can't we just hide out here?"

I laugh. "No, baby. She drove a good ways. Let's play nice."

She pushes up off her stomach and stands. I grab the blanket and shake it out as we walk toward the house.

*

"Hey, Mom," Sara says as we walk up to the porch. I see Walter, too, and I shake his hand.

"Walter, how are you doing?"

"Good, son. How are you?"

"Doing fine, thank you."

"Where did you two come from?" Debbie asks.

"We were just enjoying the sun," she says, giving her mom a hug.

"It's too hot to be out here."

"It's not hot today," Sara replies.

"Well, I guess it's a matter of opinion."

I roll my eyes when I turn my head and open the door. "After you, Debbie." I smile at the woman who is too clingy and annoys the piss out of me.

"See, you haven't done much with the place," she says, taking a seat on the couch.

"Debbie," Walter warns.

"I'm just stating facts. You need some color in this place. We can go shopping if you want, Sara."

"No thanks, Mama. Cash and I are decorating it here and there."

"Suit yourself," she says, linking her fingers on her lap.

"Would you like something to drink?" Sara asks.

"Yes, I'll take some tea."

"I don't have any made. Would water be okay?"

"You don't keep tea made here?"

"No, I don't like to get into a habit of drinking it all the time."

"You grew up drinking it all the time."

"Well, things change, Mom."

She sighs. "Water is fine."

"Would you like a beer, Walter?" I ask.

"I see you're still drinking," Debbie chimes in.

"Yep," I reply.

"A beer would be nice, son. Thank you."

I nod before Sara and then walk to the kitchen. Sara grabs at her hair as I open the fridge. "What is she even doing here?" she says in a harsh whisper.

"Guess she misses driving us fucking crazy."

Sara laughs as I hand her the water pitcher, and she fills her mom's glass.

"Guess she does," she agrees.

"You want a beer?"

"Yes, and after this visit, I'm going to need something stronger, so be ready to go out."

"Yes, ma'am," I reply. I slap her ass as I walk by and head back into the living room.

"Here you go, Mom." Sara hands her the glass, and Debbie gasps.

"What the hell did you do?" she asks in horror. I realize she is talking about her daughter's wrist, and again I curse under my breath. "When did this happen?" She looks over at me. I swallow and twist a beer cap off before handing it to Sara.

"Someone answer me, dammit."

"Mom."

"No! Don't you *Mom* me. You cut your wrist and no one tells me? I've had it. I knew something like this was going to happen. I knew you shouldn't have moved away from me. Walter, look at our baby's wrist."

Walter looks grim as he peers over at his daughter's arm. "Why didn't you call us?" he asks Sara.

"I didn't want to worry you. I had a bad moment, but I'm better, Daddy. I'm on my meds, and I'm seeing a therapist. Things are better."

He nods, but I see the worry behind his eyes. I don't blame him. If it were my daughter, I'd be worried, too. And the mention of her meds reminds me she didn't call them in.

"You should have called us the minute this happened, Cash. How are we to trust you with our child when you let something like this—"

"Stop," Sara cuts in. "Mom, I will not have you blame this on Cash. It is not his fault. It's no one's fault. I'm sick, and sometimes I get sad and I can't control it. No one can. It's just who I am. But

I'm better now. There is no need to worry, and you will not come into my home and blame my husband for something he had no part in."

Debbie huffs, and Walter stands. "We'll be on our way now."

"There's no need to leave," I say to him.

"No, son, it's getting late." He shakes my hand. Debbie stands, too, and Sara gives her a hug.

"I made the call for him to not contact you, Mom. Don't be upset with Cash."

"But why?" I hear Debbie ask.

"Because I'm not your baby anymore. I'm grown, and we have to deal with this on our own."

"You'll always be my baby." Debbie sniffs, and Sara sighs.

"I love you, Mom. Have a safe trip home."

Sara hugs her dad, and I walk them out. Debbie doesn't speak to me as she goes to the car, but Walter does. "I've always liked you…" he says, turning to face me. He slides his hands into his pockets and looks past me. "Because of the love my daughter has for you. It's as clear as the sky is blue." He sighs and looks up, but then turns his attention back to me, and I see his anger simmer behind his blue eyes. "My opinion of you will change if something happens to her on your watch. Do you hear me?"

"Yes, sir."

"Take care of her, Cash."

"I do every day," I reply.

He nods and walks to the car. I watch them leave, and I get a strong urge to ram my fist into a wall. "Fuck."

"Cash, don't let them get to you," Sara tells me.

"They don't have to," I say back to her. "*I* get to me. If I would have been there more for you, you wouldn't have tried to take your life."

"You were there for me. This wasn't about you or them. It was me."

"Why?" I ask her. "Why the fuck do you want to end your life? I don't understand it. I couldn't be happier. Why am I not enough for you?"

"You are enough. You've always been enough," she says, putting her hand on my arm. I shrug it off.

"No, if I was enough, you wouldn't have sliced your fucking wrist." She pales, and I feel like shit. I sigh and run a frustrated hand through my hair. I need to leave. I need some space, but I'm fucking terrified to leave her alone. I look over at her. "I need to take a drive. Promise me you won't do anything stupid."

"Cash."

"Fucking promise me, Sara."

"I promise," she says quietly. I nod and grab my keys. "I'll be back in a little bit."

*

I park my truck outside of Banner's and shut it off. It's not busy tonight, and I'm glad. I want to have a few drinks without anyone bothering me. It's hard being married to someone who doesn't always want to live. It's hard dealing with her mood swings, her temper, and her outbursts. It's hard dealing with the highs, and the fucking lows are going to be the death of me. Call me an asshole for bitching about this, but sometimes a man just needs a beer and a night alone. A night without worrying if his wife is going to be too sad when he gets home or if she will be walking the fucking streets because she got lonely. I push the bar door open and walk inside, noticing a few couples dancing together. I head for the bar.

"What's up, Cash? What'll you have?"

"Can I get a bottle from you?"

"A bottle?" Banner asks.

"Yeah, rough day."

"You going to have a ride home?"

"Am I the cop or are you?" I ask him. "I don't mean to sound like a dick, but just give me the damn bottle."

He narrows his eyes, but eventually shrugs. "Yes, sir."

I pay him for the bottle before I take it and my shot glasses and find a faraway booth.

Lining the shot glasses up, I fill each one then place the bottle onto the table. One by one I down the drinks, and in no time I'm piss drunk and staring at the almost empty bottle in front of me. Memories of the past flow through my mind, and I think back on the day I told my parents I was going to ask Sara to marry me.

I walk into the house and kiss my mama on the cheek. She's in her cooking apron, and the smell of bacon fills the house I grew up in. Old flower wallpaper makes up the walls in the kitchen, and her stove should have been replaced years ago, but she says, 'Just because something has a little age on it, doesn't mean you should throw it out. It still gets supper cooked, doesn't it?' Dad walks in dressed for work, and I'm glad they are both here.

"I've got some news," I say. They both turn to me, and I bounce my leg because I'm nervous. My parents like Sara okay, but they know about her issues and have expressed their feelings about it more than once. You'll always have to worry. We want you to be happy. *But they don't understand she is my happy.*

"Well, out with it, Cash," Mama says. I pull a box out of my pocket and place it onto the island. Mama gasps and Dad walks over to the coffeepot.

"I'm going to ask Sara to marry me."

Mama's eyes fill with tears, and she sighs like she has been defeated—like all the years she has tried to talk me into having a relationship with some 'normal' girl have gone to waste. It was always a pointless conversation, one that I listened to out of respect for her. But one that went in one ear and out the other. I love Sara. Period. You don't choose love; love chooses you. Once Dad fills his coffee, he walks out of the house. Mama gives me a sad smile. "He just needs some time, baby."

"Yeah," I say, grabbing the box and following my dad. "You just going to walk away?" I ask once I'm outside. He opens his car door and looks back at me.

"You'd have me do something else?"

I shrug. "I don't know, Dad. Maybe tell me congratulations. Best wishes and all that."

"Best wishes, son." He grabs his coffee from the top of his car before he gets inside. I watch him drive away, and in that moment I know I am going to be alone in this.

"Cash, son?" I hear and look from the bottle at the chief.

"Oh, look, you're here," I say. "Pull up a chair and have a few with me. Oops," I say, looking down at the bottle. "Think we may need more."

"I think you've had enough."

"I think I need just one more, though," I say, tipping the bottle up and downing the rest.

"Let me take you home."

"Home would be nice," I say as I go to stand. The floor shifts, and I close my eyes, trying to regain my balance or make my brain not shake so much. "I'm drunk," I say.

"I do believe you are. Come on. Let me help you."

I do as the chief says, and he helps me get into his car. He rolls the windows down, and I lean my head out. The night air feels good and helps to defog my cloudy brain.

"You okay?" he asks me after we're a good ways down the road.

"Been better."

"Downing a whole bottle tells me this isn't one of those better times," he says, and I notice he is taking the long way. I look out at the night sky and sigh.

"Sometimes it's hard being Sara's husband," I say more so to myself, but Drew hears me.

"Do you love her?" he asks.

"Huh?"

"Do you love her?"

"Yes."

"Well, no one said love was going to be easy, but no one tells you how damn hard it can be, either. How bad it can get at times, with bills and the loads of stress everyday life can throw at you. Unfortunately, none of us are given a handbook when we place those rings on each other's fingers, but son, if you love her, then that's all you need. You hold on to that love. You remember when she is at her worst what you love about her at her best. When she is upset, you remember how much you love her smile, so you can make her show it again. At your lowest moments, you remember your highest. Know that as long as you keep that love alive, you'll always have better days. We will never be here again. This moment will pass and one day be a distant memory, and so will every other moment in your life. So you have to decide—am I going to make this a good memory, or am I going to let this little bump in the road be a time I look back on and not smile?"

"Chief, I believe you could be a therapist, but I'm either going to puke in your car or on this old road," I say, grabbing onto the door handle. Drew slams on the brakes, and I open the door. I heave it all out and continue to do so almost all the way home.

*

I thank the chief, and now that I've gotten it all out of me, I can walk better as I make my way inside the house.

"Cash?" I hear from the couch. Sara stands up, and I sigh.

"I'm sorry, baby."

"No, I'm sorry," she says, walking over to me. I see tears in her eyes, but I stop her.

"Unless you want puke on you, let's hold off on the hugging."

"You threw up?" she asks, concerned.

"That's what happens when you down a whole bottle of whiskey. I need a shower, and then I wanna sleep this off. Can we talk tomorrow?"

"Yes, I'm just glad you're home."

"Me, too, baby. Me, too."

Chapter Eleven
Sara

The sound of birds singing outside my window wakes me, and I stretch and roll over. Cash is lying on his stomach with an open palm facing my way. I softly grab his fingers, and he feels it. His eyes open, and he winces at the sunlight coming in through the window.

"I'll close the curtains," I say. He shuts his eyes and nods. Pinching the bridge of his nose, he rolls over and the sheet falls below his waist, revealing my husband's beautiful body. Getting up, I slide the curtains closed before I sit back down on the bed.

"I'm so sorry about last night," he says. His voice is groggy, and I'm sure he feels like shit.

"Me, too. Don't worry about it, okay? I know it can all be too much sometimes."

"I shouldn't have acted that way, though."

"Cash, if you didn't go a little crazy yourself every once in a while, then I'd think you were a saint."

He chuckles. "I'm no saint, baby."

"You're pretty damn close." I lean down and kiss his hair. "Water? Headache meds?"

"Please," he says. I nod and slip off of the bed, but he grabs my hand and I turn around to face him. "I love you," he tells me.

"I'll love you crazy."

He smiles. "Maybe you do."

*

I tie off the last balloon before I grab the string and cut off another piece. My fingers ache from the fifty something balloons I've tied. I grab three and wrap them around the candy bags we have made. Leigh walks over with a glass of ice water, and I take it.

"Thanks," I tell her. I down the glass because it's hot today, and if we don't get this party started, the candy is going to melt.

"I think the kids will be happy," Maci says as she places the bags of candy onto the many tables. We're throwing a party for the kids in town. It's to give them something to do, and we encourage the parents to bring old books they no longer want so others can read them.

Maci has on big-framed sunglasses, and I wish I had brought mine. It's sunny today, and I can already feel the burn on my shoulders from being out here for over an hour.

"They should be." I look around at the bouncy house, the corn hole game, and the small tank for bobbing for apples. We've got candy, cake, ice cream, watermelon, and of course, balloons for the kids. A slip and slide is set up for the older ones, and this evening we are playing *The Goonies* on the projector and big screen we have set up. Half of these kids have probably never seen it before, but it's one of the best.

"People should start showing up soon," Maci says. "How about you be in charge of the books that get dropped off? Just write them down and who donated them, and we can send out thank you letters after this is all said and done.

"Okay."

"What can I do?" Leigh asks.

"Make sure the big kids aren't making out anywhere," Maci says.

I laugh, "Ahh, the good ol' days."

"Right? I remember when Mark and I would sneak off and make out for hours. Now, it's a quick kiss goodbye in the mornings and a glad-you're-home kiss in the evenings. Hell, I'm lucky if I get any foreplay before sex these days. It's always wham-bam-thank-you-ma'am."

I burst out laughing. "I think that's called marriage."

"What about you and Lucas?" Leigh questions Maci.

She looks over and shrugs. "Could be worse. The kids are here," she says, clearly changing the subject and walking off. Leigh passes by me as she is heading for the corn hole game.

"I wonder when she is going to stop this pretending bullshit and tell us what's going on."

"Leigh," I say.

She shrugs. "Just saying what you're thinking."

I look over at Maci as she drops some apples into the water, feeling sad for my friend and wondering why she hasn't removed those shades all morning, even when inside. I turn when I see Cash pull up in his police truck. All eyes turn to my guy, because he is gorgeous. He climbs out, and I see his brown eyes look for me. His dark hair has had his hand run through it, and I can tell he's gotten a trim. He spots me and smiles. It's heart melting and all white teeth.

"Hey, baby," I say as I walk over to him.

"Hey, y'all have outdone yourselves. It looks great out here."

"Thanks. It was a job."

He leans down and kisses my lips, and I smile against his.

"Get a room," Leigh calls out, and we laugh.

"How are the Kingsleys?" I ask as we walk hand in hand.

"Same as always. This morning, Elizabeth said she was making coffee and asked Joe if he wanted any. He said no, so she only made enough for herself. He then changed his mind after the coffee was made. He got mad at her and told her that after ten years of marriage she should know how wishy-washy he is and that she should have made more just in case. She then said she doesn't like to waste things, so he should have been sure. He got even more pissed, saying she wastes things all the time, and then he grabbed the coffeemaker and tossed it outside. It broke against the road, and she started crying and saying her mama gave her that as a wedding gift. She went and got the keys to his lawnmower. Now, get this, baby," Cash tells me as he leans in. "The woman cranked the thing and drove it straight into the pond!"

"Really?" I ask, wide-eyed.

"Really," he says.

"What happened then?"

"Then I had to take Joe in."

"Why?"

"Because he was so damn mad, he told me to put the handcuffs on him or he was going to choke her to death."

I laugh because I just can't help it. "My God, those two."

"I know. Promise me we won't get like that."

"Promise, promise," I say, shaking my head and grinning.

*

The day passes with water balloon fights and soaked faces from bobbing for apples. The slip and slide got torn, and the bouncy house was so wet no one could stand up in it anymore. We've cleaned up most of everything, and as the sun starts to say goodbye, we lay out blankets and I pass out popcorn. We've got a pile of books to label tomorrow, and I look over at Maci who still wears her glasses. She loads the books into a wagon, and I follow.

"It was a good day, wasn't it?"

"It was a perfect day."

"Too bad Lucas couldn't make it out here," I say,

"Yeah," she says quietly.

"Want me to help you unload these?"

"No, you go enjoy the movie with Cash. I'll probably get to these tomorrow."

"Okay," I say, still looking at her. She walks over to the computer, and I watch to see if she is going to remove her shades.

She looks my way. "Anything else?"

I sigh. "Are you going to keep those on all night?"

"What?"

"Your glasses."

"Oh, I forgot I even had them on," she lies and still doesn't take them off.

"Maci," I say.

"I'll see you tomorrow," she says. "Thanks for your help today." She hurries to the back before I can get another word in. I sigh and walk back out to the movie. Cash sits on a blanket up against a tree, and I make my way over.

"Where'd you go?" he asks as I get on my knees and move myself in between his legs. I lean back on his chest and look toward the screen.

“I went to check on Maci.”

“Everything okay?” he asks me.

“I’m not sure.”

“Can I help?”

“I’ll let you know.”

*

A soft wind blows around me as I sit in the field behind our house. My hair tickles my face, and I move it to the side. It’s long, and for some reason today, it’s driving me nuts, but today seems off anyway. I look through my journal and see that for the most part my moods have been pretty regular. No shifty thoughts lately. I flip to a clean page and in big letters I write, TODAY I’M CUTTING MY HAIR!

I stand and grab the blanket I was sitting on and walk the short distance back to the house. Hanging the blanket over the porch railing, I walk into the house, noticing the screen door still has a hole in it. This is getting old, and I’m tired of killing flies, but first things first. I walk upstairs to the bathroom and grab the scissors Cash uses to trim his beard. Hair be gone. I look at it in the mirror before I hold up a piece, and in one move I cut it. I watch it fall to the floor before I look back up at my reflection. Chop, chop. It goes as easy as butter spreading on a hot piece of bread. I cut around until it is up to my shoulders, and even then I cut some more. After I'm satisfied, I toss the scissors back into the basket and run downstairs to grab the broom.

After I sweep up the hair, I grab the keys. Cash has been leaving Old Blue here now that the chief lets him take the police truck home. I start up the truck and make my way to the hardware store.

*

"Sara," Mark greets. "New hairdo?"

"Yep, I decided I wanted it shorter. I'm here to buy a new screen door."

"You don't wanna just replace the screen?" he asks.

"Nope, I want a new door."

He shrugs. "All right, right this way."

*

After I leave the store with my new screen door and a shitload more flowers, I make my way back home. I pull up to the house and lift the tailgate down. Grabbing the door, I head to the porch and lean it against the railing. Walking inside, I look for a screwdriver in the cabinets above the washing machine. I unscrew the old door and get started on the new one. It's not easy to do because I have to hold it up while I secure the screws, but I get it, and after a bit I've got a brand new door. I open and shut it a few times to make sure it's screwed in tight. Once I'm satisfied, I take the old door and load it onto the back of the truck and get to work on my flowers.

*

Cash

"I'll see you in the morning, Anne."

"Have a good night." She smiles as I push the door open and the bell rings above me. A commotion causes my eyes to divert to Banner's Bar down the road, and I see Lucas' truck parked there. He stumbles out of the door.

"I don't want your fucking liquor anyway," he yells, almost tripping over his own feet. He's drunk, and anyone watching this can tell. I climb into my truck and ride down that way. Turning my blue lights on, I park behind his vehicle so he can't get out.

"Well, well, if it isn't the boy in blue."

"Lucas." I nod as I step out of my truck.

"You good here?" Banner asks me.

"I've got it. Thanks, man."

Banner nods before he shuts the door. "There's no reason for you to be down here. You just go on about your way," Lucas slurs, and I roll my eyes.

"Don't think so. You're drunk, and I can't have you driving around."

He laughs. "Since when you think you're in charge of my driving, buddy?"

"Don't make a scene. Just get into my truck and let me take you home."

"I don't think I want to ride with you."

"You don't have a choice."

"Oh, I don't, do I?"

"No, you either ride with me or I can handcuff you and take you down to the station. Which is it…*buddy*?"

He narrows his eyes at me and sucks his teeth. "Fine, deputy. I'll let you give me a ride home." I climb into my truck as he gets into the back, and I put it in drive. "Your little wife still having issues with panic attacks?" he asks. I look in the rearview mirror at him. He's leaned back and looking out the window. His eyes are shiny red, and they have that unclear look in them. I don't respond.

"You know, Maci used to get those when we were pregnant, but that was a while ago," he tells me as he lifts his hat on his head. He leaves it sitting on top of his hair, and I see a flash of something come across his face. Regret maybe? I fix my eyes back on the road and adjust my own hat as we pull out of downtown and onto the road to his house. The man who makes my fingers twitch keeps sucking his teeth, and I want him out of my truck.

"You think she might try to slit her wrist again? I heard about that. Gotta be rough dealing with someone who would rather try to kill herself than live with you."

I slam on the brakes and throw the gear shifter in park. Jumping out, I round the vehicle and swing open his door. I grab a fistful of his shirt and yank him out. He falls to the ground, but I lift him up and throw him against my truck. He holds up his hands and lets a laugh out. "You piece of shit," I say, shoving him again. He stumbles, and his knees give out. "Get up." He doesn't. He just rolls onto his back and laughs harder. "Get the fuck up!"

"Come on, deputy. I didn't mean to get you all riled up," he says, putting his palms down flat on the rough gravel. I see pieces of rock fall from his palms as he tries to push his drunk ass up but fails. It takes everything in me to not kick his sorry ass, but I notice how drunk he is and I see what he is trying to do.

"Get in the fucking truck," I say, leaving him on the ground. I spit as I round the corner and jump back into my seat. I slam the door, and once the asshole is back in, I press the gas, catching a wheel and throwing black smoke and pieces of gravel into the air.

Once I'm at his house, I get out and open his door. He's passed out. "Shit." I don't want to carry his ass, but I guess I don't have a choice. I see Maci standing on the porch, and I lean down and lift the man over my shoulder. Walking up onto the porch, Maci quickly heads over to the door and opens it for me, and I toss him onto the couch.

"You going to be okay with him?" I ask her. I turn around, and that's when I see it. It's barley there, but gray mixed with black lines her left eye. "Did he hit you?" She turns her face so I can't see. I look at her cheeks as they turn red and she fidgets.

"I ran into the dang door. I wasn't paying attention." She waves her hand dismissively. Lucas makes a noise, and I look back at him.

"Maci, if he is hitting you, you don't have to stay here. We can get you help."

"No, it's not that. I'm just clumsy sometimes. I better get him taken care of. Thanks for bringing him home, Cash. I really appreciate it."

"Are you sure you're okay?"

"Yes, I'm good. Really."

I search her face, knowing she is lying to me, but if she doesn't verbally tell me, and I don't see it myself, there isn't anything I can do about it. She walks over to the door and stands beside it after she pulls it open. I take this as my cue to leave.

"Okay. Let us know if you need anything."

"I will. Thanks again."

I walk out of the house with a bad feeling in my chest. That asshole is hitting her.

*

Pulling up to the yard, I see Sara outside. I squint from the sun and look toward her as she stands. Her blonde hair has been seriously chopped off, but she smiles like nothing has changed. More flowers have been added to her garden, and she wipes her knees off before she walks over to me.

"What happened to your hair?" I ask as she stands on her tippy toes and kisses me.

"It was getting in my way."

"Couldn't pull it back?"

"Nope, I wanted a change," she answers. I narrow my eyes. "Stop looking at me like that." She's hands on her hips and red on her shoulders.

"Baby."

"Don't baby me." She walks back to the garden and starts cleaning up her things. I notice only half the flowers are planted. "You don't like it?" she asks.

"You'd look good with no hair. It's just a drastic quick change."

"Not really."

"Yes, really."

She sighs and fills her hands with too much.

"Give me some of that."

"I've got it," she fires back. I watch her walk to the porch before I follow.

"Have you been feeling okay?"

"Seriously not this again." She drops her stuff and yanks the—what I see now is a new screen door—open. My girl has been busy.

"New door?" I question with a lift of my brow.

"Yeah, I asked you to fix it and you didn't, so I did."

"Sorry, I've just been busy."

"It's fine, Cash. I can take care of some things by myself."

"I didn't say you couldn't."

"Once again you didn't have to. Your actions show me that you think I can't handle anything by myself."

"How, Sara?"

"You baby me."

"How?"

"You just do."

"Tell me how I do it and I'll stop."

"For one, every time I do anything spur of the moment, you think it's more than it is. Sometimes people just do things, Cash," she says, walking into the dining room. I see the furniture has been changed around, but the things on the hutch have not been put back up. She grabs the dusting spray and an old rag. She quickly sprays and wipes, sprays and wipes. I don't take my eyes off of her. Leaning against the doorframe, I cross my arms and watch my high girl. She doesn't even realize that she is, but I see it. I see the change in her eyes, and I can tell her mind is running a mile a minute.

"So, I just ignore the fact you went to the hardware store and bought a shitload more flowers you didn't really need? I should ignore the fact you went and bought a new door when you could have just gotten some new screen? I should ignore the fact that you fucking chopped your damn hair off?"

She turns to me and sighs. "I wanted a haircut, so I cut it." She tosses the rag onto the table and starts putting things back on the shelf. "I wanted a new door, so I bought one. I wanted more fucking flowers, so I got them. End of."

"Fine. I'm done talking about this anyway." I throw my hands up because this isn't a winning battle. Sara is on a one-track mindset right now, and I have no say.

"Good," she says, but she doesn't look back at me. She continues to place the picture frames and whatnots up.

"Good," I say back before I walk toward the stairs.

*

I grab a towel and wrap it around my waist. Water drops from my hair, and I run a hand through it. Fucking baby pisses me off. How can she not see all of those things were irrational and should have been talked about? She spent God knows how much on all those flowers, and she chopped all her hair off. I open the bathroom door, and my eyes land on her as she sits on the floor. She's only in a tank top and black boy shorts, and I can't be pissed at her anymore. She's leaning against the wall with her journal in her hand and tears in her pretty eyes. She looks up, and the tears fall.

"Why are you crying?"

"You know I just cry sometimes." She shrugs, and I walk over to her. "I'm sorry," she mumbles. I sigh and reach my hand out.

"Come here." She looks up at my hand and our palms touch before I link our fingers together. "Are you okay?" I ask her as I sit down on the bed and she stands between my knees. Baby blue eyes are filled with tears, but she gives me a small smile as she looks down at my bare chest.

"I'm okay." She leans down and kisses my forehead. Picking up my hand, she places it on her ass. "Make me feel good," she whispers to me. "Make me shut down for a minute."

I grab a handful and pull her closer to me. The anger I had earlier from drunk ass and the way she presses my buttons come to my mind, and I reach my hand up and grab the back of her neck, pulling her face down to mine. I kiss her roughly. She opens her mouth, letting my tongue enter, and I grip her skin tighter.

In one swift move, I switch places with her, letting my towel fall. She opens her knees, and I climb in between, quickly moving her boy shorts down her legs. I press forward and spread her legs farther apart. My dick slides against her, and I don't even have to test that she is ready. I push inside, and her eyes close. She grabs the blanket, and her mouth hangs open as I love her. Taking out all the pent-up anger she ignites inside of me, I rare back and slam forward, over and over again until she is nothing but fists full of sheets and I'm just a man sick in love, falling from a high Sara can only give me.

Chapter Twelve
Sara

My fingertips lightly tap, and the coolness they feel from the crystal clear water makes me hesitant to jump in, so I dip my feet instead. "Drinks!" Leigh shouts as she walks out onto the patio. I grab mine, and Maci does the same. "To hot summers with cool chicks." Leigh smiles.

"What she said," Maci says before taking a sip of her drink. Ice clinks the side of my glass, and I lick the salt from my lips.

"Wait. I didn't even think about it, but should you be drinking with your medication?" Maci asks me.

"Probably not." I shrug before I take another sip. She shakes her head at me.

"What?" I ask.

"Just don't think it's a good idea, is all."

"Oh, leave her alone, Maci. Let the girl have some fun." Leigh puts her drink down and reaches on the other side of the pool for her float with the bug net. Maci removes her shoes and slides her socks off. I see a bruise on her leg, but I look away. She could have just run into a piece of furniture. I do it all the time. My hip has a bruise on it now because my brain can't remember where the bedpost is.

Leigh screams when she tips over on her float, and Maci and I laugh when she comes back up. Wet brown hair covers her face, and she huffs. "Man, I didn't wanna get my damn hair wet. Now I gotta wash it again for date night with Mark."

"Date night?" I ask, waiting for details.

"Yep. Mark is taking me to see a movie."

"Sweet," I say. Leigh regains her balance on the float and takes hold of the edge of the pool so she can grab her drink.

"Well, it's the least he can do," she says.

"Why do you say that?" Maci asks.

"'Cause I, you know what, in his truck today."

"What?" Maci says.

"You know," Leigh repeats with a quirky lift of her brow.

"I seriously don't." Maci looks over at me, and I grin.

"I think she means a blow job."

Maci scrunches her face. "Gross, Leigh."

"What? Sometimes you gotta do what you gotta do to keep the ol' husband happy."

"Yeah, but your husband is friendly Mark."

"He's friendly all right." Leigh winks, and I laugh again.

"But for real. You can't tell me you've never given Lucas a blow job."

"Not in a car."

"What about you, Sara? Cash get any fun action out of you in a car before?"

I bite my lip and look down at the water. After prom night, Cash and I could hardly keep our hands off of each other. I remember the smell of his mom's air freshener hanging from the rearview mirror. Cash took us down to Lake Side, and we parked the car and got in the back seat. His hands were all over me and anywhere else they could fit. Our lips were like magnets, drawn to each other and hard to break apart. He kissed every inch of my body that night, and I remember thinking this is what love is. This feeling in my chest when I hear his name. These crazy emotions of not knowing if I want to laugh or cry because he makes me so damn happy. The desperate need to feel him and have him near me as much as possible.

"I'll take that blush as a yes," Leigh says, and I notice her and Maci looking at me.

"You're lucky to find someone you love so deeply and they return that love just as much," Maci says. I give her a small smile before I take a sip of my drink.

I didn't fall in love with Cash. It was something that happened slowly, like a vine growing up a fencepost. We were so young when we met that I hardly remember a time when I didn't know him…

The school bell rang, and the sound of kids jumping up from their desks echoed through the classrooms, while laughter and loud mouths filled the wide hallways. I still remember the smell of cigarette smoke coming from the girls' bathroom. The sounds of my science teacher's heels against the hard tile floor. Coach Dudley's short shorts as he walked through the maze of excited-to-be-out-of-school kids with a big smile on his face because he was on summer vacation, too.

I walked up to my group of friends just like any other day, but it wasn't any other day. Cash leaned against the wall, one knee bent and his foot flat on the brick his back rested on, while the other was planted firmly on the ground. He was slightly smirking at something one of his friends was saying. His hand was slid into his jeans pocket, while his books were carelessly stacked on the ground beside his leg. I walked up, his eyes looked to me, and that's the moment I fell for him. I don't know why. It was something about the way he looked at me, like he saw me for me. Not the quirky, popular girl who was weird sometimes. He saw the girl who was confused with her emotions, the girl who cried behind closed doors and one day felt no need to get out of bed. He saw me—the actress without her lines. After that, I was nervous around him and got butterflies, but I didn't tell anyone because this was Cash—sweet guy, cuter than all the rest, and my friend.

But soon, he started asking me if I wanted to grab a bite to eat, just the two of us, without our friends. He asked me if I wanted him to carry my books or if I wanted to keep some things in his locker so I wouldn't have to walk all the way to mine because all my classes were closer to his. Sometimes he put his arm around me or brushed his hand against mine. Little shows of affection here and there. Then one day, after a night of hanging out at Lake Side and a stomach full of beer, he grabbed my hand and told me he wanted to show me something. We walked away from our friends, and he took me around the backside of an abandoned building. I was laughing at something, and then all of a sudden he pressed me up against the wall. My lungs stopped taking in air, and I felt swarms of butterflies in my belly. He told me he wanted to kiss me, and I let him. I let him kiss me in the moonlight up against an old building with our friends' laughter in the background, and it was the best kiss I'd ever had.

*

The sound of the ball hitting the metal bat echoes in the air, and I stand up, clapping my hands excitedly as Cash runs. Leigh sits beside me—gum chewing, baseball hat on her head with her brown hair pulled through the back. I've gone and had my hair fixed, and now I've got a Meg Ryan look going on. It's short, and I love it. I look back at the cars parked and see Maci walking up with her new habit between her fingers. Smoke blows from her mouth as I give her a wave, letting her know where we are. She flicks the cigarette and turns her head away so not to blow smoke in anyone's face. She sits down beside me, and I look over at her. "You know smoking is really bad for you."

"Just like drinking with your meds, huh?" she says.

I lift my brow and smile a little. "Touché, my friend. Touché."

"Where's Lucas?" Leigh asks.

"Lucas is passed out, so I figured why am I going to sit at home?"

My friend just started smoking, and her husband isn't treating her any better. It's not a secret that I'm worried—I've told her more than once. Her carefree attitude is understandable, but it doesn't distract me from the bruises on her arms. She sees me looking and gives me a glare.

"I'm not going to say anything," I say as I look back toward the field and see Cash on third base. Two more runs and we will win this.

"You know I don't crawl in the fetal position and take it, don't you?" This is the first time she has ever acknowledged him hitting her. I don't say anything—too scared she won't continue.

"I'm filing for divorce. Give me some of that gum," she says to Leigh who also has a look of *what the hell?*

"Both of you stop."

She grabs a handful of Big League Chew and takes her shades off. I see a small shade of blue under her eye. It's fresh because I saw her yesterday, and it wasn't there.

"His drinking is getting out of hand, and his hand is getting braver. I'm sick of it, and I'm going to end up smothering him in his sleep if he doesn't kill me first."

I look around at the other people on the bleachers. A woman looks our way with a shocked face.

"Turn around, Gladys Kravitz," Leigh says, and I try to hold my laugh in. Maci doesn't, and Leigh snickers with her.

"I'm going to need yours and Cash's help," Maci says after the giggles stop and her face turns serious.

"This man isn't going to let me go without a fight." She looks off, and a crease forms between her brows. Her eyes fill with unshed tears she doesn't even seem to know are there.

"He wasn't always like this, and it breaks my damn heart," she says quietly, and there's the friend I know and have come to love. She sniffs and straightens her back. "But people change, things change, and as much as you want them to stay the same, it just isn't always the case." She looks down at her fingers and sighs. I look out at the field and see that Cash has already run home and so has the other player. We won, and I didn't even notice.

"We are here for you. Whatever you need," I tell her.

*

I'd tell you I was a pro at driving the motorcycle, but I'd be lying. Cash is, though, so we head out of town with a blanket and a picnic basket. Cotton candy skies are above us as the sun decides to stretch its light and wake up for the day. It's early morning, and the wind against my face is cool. I feel okay today. I haven't been taking my medicine like I should, though, because I'm tired of how sleepy it makes me.

*

Cash slows the bike down and comes to a complete stop. I hop off first and remove my helmet. I run a hand through my hair and look out at the view. The sun shines brightly now, making a layer of gold flakes across the water. The blue diving board I jumped off of more times than I can count rests in the middle of the lake on a platform, and the sound of water lapping against the dock I remember being bigger is the only thing that can be heard. It's peaceful out here, but it used to be full of splish-splashing and laughing kids, drunk teenagers, and late night bonfires. I look over at my husband and smile.

"Wanna go for a dip?" he asks me. My grin widens, and I squeal when Cash takes off running and I do the same. He pulls his shirt up from behind his neck, and I grab mine from the bottom and toss it behind me. Our feet knock against the dock. He yells, "cannon ball" before he disappears into the water with a big splash. Jumping up, I toss my hands into the air and leap. It almost feels like flying until cold water touches my toes. The loud noise of our splash mutes, and then darkness and the rushing of water surround me as bubbles bubble up. A light feeling of weightlessness takes over me. My arms go limp, and my neck rests back. I hold my breath and enjoy this quick moment of being totally alone under a space so big. It's tranquility and awe at the same time. I feel his hands under my arms before I am forced to the top. I let air rush into my lungs as Cash moves my hair out of my face.

"What the hell are you doing?"

"Just shutting out the noise for a second."

Brown eyes and messy hair looks at me. He doesn't understand. He wants to, but he just can't. I splash him and grin as I take off back toward the dock.

*

We lie on the blanket, soaking up some rays and eating the fruit I packed.

"You miss this place?" Cash asks me. I lean back on my arms and look around me.

"I miss the moments we had here."

"Yeah, me, too," he agrees.

"Remember when Sky and Johnathan got pretend married out on the dock?"

"Yep. She had on her mother's old wedding dress, and they jumped into the water after. She was grounded for a month." I laugh, remembering how brown the dress was when she got out of the water.

"Over there is where I first kissed you," he says.

"And it was the best kiss I'd ever had."

"I hope you didn't have many."

"Nope, that's why it was the best." I grin, nudging him. He rolls his eyes.

"You planning on seeing your parents while we're here?" I ask.

He looks down and shakes his head. "Nah." I look away and watch a flock of ducks fly over the lake. Cash and his parents haven't spoken in a while. He doesn't think I know, but I realize they weren't too happy with his decision to marry me. I was too messed up for the sheriff's boy. I am messed up, but we make it work.

*

After we let the sun dry us, we get back on the bike and drive down some roads that haven't had our tires on them in more than a while. Sunlight does its best to shine through the woods, but the trees are thick. I wrap my arms around Cash's waist, wishing I could kiss his neck, but these dang helmets are in the way. We head into town just to ride by the old grocery store parking lot where we all used to hang out. No cars are there now, but on the weekends and sometimes after school, it was packed and everyone walked from car to car talking and cutting up. Nothing else to do in a small town. We circle back and head toward what we now call home.

Chapter Thirteen
Sara

I sniff and a sneeze comes out worse than the one before. “Bless you,” Maci yells from somewhere I have no idea. It’s cleaning day at the library, and I’ve never seen so much dust.

“When is the last time you did this?” I yell back.

“Last summer.”

I turn when I see her standing in the row I’m seated in. Her red hair is piled up, and like always she wears jeans and a blouse. She laughs at my makeshift facemask. It’s an old rag with loose strings, which just so happens to fit perfectly behind my ears.

“Don’t laugh. I’m just trying to prevent a major sinus infection.”

“Well, from the way you’ve been sneezing, I don’t think it’s working.”

I remove it. “I think you’re right.” I sigh and run a hand through my hair. I hear the library door open, and Maci looks that way. Her eyes grow wide, and I see her swallow. I stand.

"What the fuck is this?" I hear and walk closer to Maci and see Lucas. He looks from her to me and then back to her.

"Lucas, I need you to leave."

"Leave?" he says. "I'm gone for two days working, and I come home to fucking divorce papers? Where is all of your shit, Maci?"

"Don't worry about that," she says. I can see how tired of this she really is. He walks closer to her, but she doesn't move. Either she isn't scared or she just doesn't give a shit anymore. I think it's both. He looks mad, crazy in fact, and I can smell alcohol on him from here.

He looks over at me. "You got something to do with this?"

"Leave her out of it." Maci turns to me. "Sara, go on home. I'll call you in a little bit."

"No," I say. "I'm not leaving you."

"You think you can protect her or something?"

"I think that if you try anything, you'll know we were there."

He laughs and shakes his head. Tossing the papers down, he gets in her face. "This isn't over. You know I'm not letting you go." His eyes search hers. Lucas reaches his hand up, and I see her flinch when he runs a finger down the side of her face to her neck. "I'm never letting you go." He steps on the papers and turns to leave. Once the door shuts, Maci lets out a big breath of air I had no idea she was holding. She leans down and picks up the papers before looking over at me. Tears are in her eyes, and she glances back toward the door.

"What happened?" she asks no one. "When did everything go to shit?"

*

I'm porch swinging with a beer between my legs, waiting for Cash to pull up. It's hot out, but a good breeze blows, making it more bearable. I mindlessly pick at the label on my beer and wipe the condensation on my forehead from the bottle. I hear Cash's truck, and I get up off the swing. He puts it in park, and I walk out to him.

"Got one of those for me?" He smiles.

"I've cleaned the fridge and filled it only with beer. Figure the drunkenness will take our mind off of our worries and the fact that we are starving." I smile, and he laughs.

"Who needs food anyway?"

"Right?" I say, handing him my beer. He takes a sip, and we walk onto the porch. "Maci served Lucas the divorce papers."

"Oh, yeah?" He opens the door, and I walk in first.

"Yeah, he came up to the library today."

Cash looks over at me as he removes his ball cap and hangs it by the door.

"And?"

"And he told her he wasn't letting her go."

"Where is she?"

"She's staying at her mom's house."

"She safe there?"

"I guess."

"I talked to the chief about this earlier. He said Lucas used to be a standup guy. Played football in high school. Got into a little trouble like most teens, some fights here and there, but never acted like this."

"I'm scared to ask Maci, but I wonder if he had anything to do with them losing her child."

"That's a good question," he says. Cash's new cell phone rings, and he slides it out of his pocket. "Drew?" His eyes lock on mine.

"What?" I ask.

"Yes, sir. Headed over there now." He grabs his keys from the table and hangs up.

"What is it, Cash?"

"Maci wasn't safe."

*

Cash

I pull up to Lucas' house. Leaving my lights on, I hop out of my truck and call out to Lucas.

"Lucas, it's Cash. Just come on out of the house."

I hear a scream, but it's muffled, and my heart jumps. Shit, that's Maci. Lights come up behind me, and I see it's the chief and Deputy Guzman.

"Where is he, son?" Rogers asks once he exits his truck.

"Inside, I'm guessing, and he has Maci with him. I heard her."

"He's armed," the chief says.

"What's he planning on doing here?" Guzman asks.

"I don't have a good feeling about this. Her mom called me, said he showed up over at their house with a gun. Said he'd shoot her right there if she didn't come with him. He broke their front door." Drew walks over to his truck, and I shake my head.

"Jesus," I say under my breath.

The chief gets on his microphone. "Lucas, son. Just come on out here. We just wanna talk about this." He turns to Guzman and me. "Williams, you go around back. Stay low. Guzman, you get to the side of the front porch."

I watch Guzman head to the side of the house, and once he is there, he creeps his way to the side of the porch. I quietly make my way around. I look at the chief before I disappear to the back, putting a hand over my gun.

"Lucas, this is the chief. Now come on out here, boy. Let Maci go and let's talk about this."

"I don't want to fucking talk. There is nothing to talk about!" Lucas yells from inside the house. "You boys just go on home now."

I move through overgrown grass until I reach the back door.

"Let Maci and me be. We're just going to pack up some things and head on out of here. You won't see us again."

As softly as I can, I turn the doorknob, and the door clicks open. From my memory of the house, it's not directly out of the living room, so they shouldn't hear me. I take a peek inside and hear Maci talking. "Lucas, please. What have you done? What happened to you?" she asks, and I know we need to hurry and get her out of this situation. I open the door more until I can slide inside, and I hear the chief again.

"Lucas, we don't want anyone to get hurt. Please, son, let Maci go and come on out of the house."

I look to my left and then to the right as I hear his footsteps going back and forth against the carpet. I tilt my head forward, trying to look into the living room. Maci comes into view and sees me. Her eyes go wide, and I put my finger over my lips. Her reaction goes unnoticed by Lucas, and I walk to the end of the hallway until I'm right at the edge. He paces back and forth with the gun in his hand. From here I can tell he is soaked with sweat and at least a bottle in. He puts the side of the gun to his forehead and taps it. The chief continues to talk, and Lucas pulls at his hair before he walks to the kitchen.

Adrenaline pushes through my veins, and as Lucas turns his back on me, I run as fast as I can, knocking his gun out of his hand first and then slamming him face forward to the floor. He struggles, but he's drunk and sloppy. His sharp elbow slams into my stomach, and I wince before my fist connects hard with his ribs. He hollers, and I smell the alcohol on him. I get one hand cuffed and then the other before I jump up and then yank him up, too. Maci cries, and I call out to the boys.

"Why, Lucas?" Maci continues to sob. He shakes his head with a look of pure understanding. He knows he's going away for a while. He knows he messed up.

"I'm lost," he says quietly. His face sobers, and he hangs his head as the chief and Guzman walk in.

"I've got him," Rogers says as he grabs him from the back and walks him out the door. I look over at Maci. Her face is in her hands, and she sniffs as she rubs her palms down, dropping her hands onto her lap. She looks up at me.

"Are you okay?" I ask her.

Her lips go straight, and she takes a shaky breath. "My other half just changed both of our lives without any regard of me. He turned into a person I've never met before. He pushed me around, spoke to me as though I was worthless. Not like his wife, not like the woman he has loved for years. Not like he *is* my other half. So, no, Cash, I'm not okay. I'm not going to be okay for a while." She looks past me at the wall and stands. I watch her go into the kitchen, and I don't blame her as she grabs the liquor bottle. She tosses it back and takes two big gulps without even a wince. She shakes her head. "One day I will be again, though. I will be okay again," she says it as if she is trying to convince herself.

When I walk out of the house, I'm more than positive, Maci will be okay. It may take a long time, but one day she'll be able to breathe a little better than before. She'll feel lighter, and the world won't seem so shitty. One day.

*

Sara

When I was no taller than a dog on four legs, my daddy taught me how to ride a bike. I remember this time so clearly, even though I was just five. He ran alongside me, helping me balance and making sure I didn't fall. He said it would get easier the more I did it.

"That's with everything in life, Sara. The more you do it, the easier it will be."

I did learn to ride that bike, and every time I did it, the easier it got. I got a bigger bike, and eventually, I spread my arms out wide. Sometimes I'd even get brave and close my eyes. The breeze swept over my skin, tickling my tiny arm hairs and running its fingers through my wild dirty blonde curls. I'd laugh and pretend I was no longer on a bike, but a feather, traveling to some place only the wind knew.

Unfortunately, though, my daddy was wrong. Not everything applies to that saying. Grief doesn't get easier, nor do heartache and sickness. I'm sure there are plenty of other things that are also just as hard as the first time you do them. Take my illness, for example. The more it appears, the harder the lines on my husband's face show. It never gets easier to handle. None of it.

*

You know that perfect moment right before darkness takes over the sky? There's no sun in sight, but the sky is still lightly lit, a sweet blue. I place my feet up on the edge of the porch rail and lean my head back. Taking my first sip of the icy cold beer in my hand, I lick my lips when the taste of lime hits my tongue. The clouds roll in front of the moon, getting shifted along from the wind. The leaves in the big tree ruffle from the light breeze that moves in from the field, running over my body and giving me chills that make the hair on the back of my neck stand up. My thoughts are my own. No one is here to judge me. No one even knows I sit on my front porch but the fireflies that dance in our front yard. This is what life is about. Simple moments. Quiet pieces within an hour of the twenty-four. I wish I could put this moment in a bottle, and every time things get to be too much, I can open that bottle and once again feel like I do now. Content and simply happy.

Chapter Fourteen
Cash

The bathroom floor is covered in plastic sheets that already have tiny speckles of pale yellow paint on them. Music plays from the record player in the hallway, and with her paintbrush, Sara sings and laughs. She's happy today. She's been happy for a few days now. Her hair is growing out, and I'm glad. I miss her pretty long curls. I run my paintbrush along the crown molding and am careful not to get any white paint on her yellow.

"Cash, will you slide that closer to me?"

I do as she asks, placing the paint can closer to her. I feel cold paint touch my forehead, and she giggles.

"Did you just put paint on me?" I ask.

"Just a little." She grins when I look up, and she taps her paintbrush on my nose. She laughs like it's the funniest thing ever, and I stare at her, open-mouthed.

"You better hope that comes off."

"A little paint never hurt anyone," she says before she turns her back to me and continues painting above the windowsill. She can hardly reach it, and her shirt rides up, revealing her tan skin. I dip my finger into the paint and run it from one side of her hip to the other. She sucks in air. "Cash!" She turns around and looks at me.

"A little paint never hurt anyone. Remember, baby?" I say with a smug smile before I dip my finger again. She looks from my finger to my face.

"And what do you think you're gonna do with that?"

I shrug. "I don't know just yet. But I do think a little paint on your nose wouldn't be such a bad thing."

"Oh no, you don't," she says, dropping her brush into the tub. She holds her hands out in front of her. "Put the finger down, Cash." I poke it at her. Some paint drops off my finger into the tub, landing right on her toe. I laugh.

"Cash Williams, you put that finger down and let me out of here." She's all smiles, but trying to sound serious. I climb into the tub with her and watch as she backs up. She laughs and jumps around me, out of the tub, and exits the bathroom. I follow, chasing her down the stairs. She bolts out the door onto the porch and laughs as she stands in the yard.

"What are you laughing at?" I ask.

"Your yellow nose, duh," she answers. I walk toward her. "Cash, I don't want a yellow nose."

"Well, too bad. We are teammates, and if one teammate has a yellow nose, then the other should, too."

"I don't think I wanna be your teammate then."

"This crushes me." I put a hand over my heart.

She laughs loud. "You're such a baby."

I walk closer, and she backs up. "Where exactly are you going?" I ask.

"I'll run until I can't anymore." She grins and runs a hand through her hair, removing it from her face. A huge wood bee buzzes by, and she swipes it away. I take this opportunity and grab her up. "Cash!" she yells and laughs, and I gently place her on the ground, sitting on top of her but careful not to squish her tiny body. The paint on my finger is almost dry, but I still touch her nose, even though she wiggles like a fish out of water. Her eyes are shut tight, and she has her mouth closed, but she still laughs from her chest. Her nose is now yellow like mine, and I sit back.

"Now, that's better," I say. She slaps my chest.

"Cash Williams, this paint better come off!"

"Well, you had no thought of that when you did it to me."

"That's because you're a big butthead who deserves to have a yellow nose. You're a bully, Cash."

"I am not." I smile and lean down, taking her lips with mine and making her forget what she was even saying. I taste her tongue when she opens her lips, and I rest my arms beside her head, gripping onto the just cut grass. Her fingers run over my back, and she pulls me closer, spreading her legs and letting me sink. She moans when I push forward. Just then we hear a car pull up. I open my eyes and see hers are wide. "Seems we have company," I whisper.

"Get up, you big bully." She grins, and I sit back and pull her up, too. I turn to see Chief Rogers and Anne. He opens the car door, and I look at Anne as she gets out.

"Hope we weren't interrupting anything," Drew says, clearing his throat.

"Well, of course we were, dear. Those two were about to get it on in the middle of the yard."

I laugh, and Sara blushes. "Nah, I would have taken it inside." I wink down at Sara who shakes her head at me and playfully slaps my arm.

"You two want a drink or something?" Sara asks.

"We just wanted to ride out here and tell you guys there's an amusement park just outside of town. Thought you two might enjoy that. We could have called, of course—" Anne says, blushing herself.

"But we wanted to take a drive," Drew cuts in. "And we don't know why we haven't told you two sooner about it. Anne and I used to go there all the time when we were younger."

I look down at Sara. "Wanna go have some fun?"

"Sure." She smiles.

"Umm, Cash, son, it looks like both of you got a little paint on your faces," Drew says.

Baby and I look at each other, and neither of us can help the laugh that bubbles up from our chests and bursts out of our mouths.

*

The sounds of rollercoasters swooshing through the wind and people laughing and screaming ring in my ears, and I grab Sara's hand as we walk on the black pavement.

“What do you want to ride first?” I ask her.

“Everything.” She grins big. We jump on the first ride we see. It’s a train coaster, but from the looks of it, it hauls ass and seems fun. We walk up to the line of people and stand and wait. TVs play in all corners of the line, and fans blow, giving us a little break from the heat of the day. Our turn is next. As soon as the train stops, Sara climbs in first, and I pull the bar close to us. People stand on a wooden platform and watch us, and the person operating the ride says a few safety words before he hits a green button and the ride starts. It’s slow at first, but picks up speed quickly, and before we know it, we’re flying through twists and turns. The sound of Sara’s laugh makes me smile, and she throws her hands up when we drop down a huge hill into a dark tunnel. The ride jerks sideways, surprising the hell out of me because we can’t see anything. Sara’s hands are forced down, and when we come out of the tunnel and stop, she laughs. “Holy hell, that was fun.”

*

Windblown hair and tired feet, we’ve walked all over this park and ridden everything. We’ve eaten, and I’ve played a few games, winning Sara some stuffed animals, which she gives away to the kids except a little elephant. “I love elephants,” she says.

“I love you,” I tell her.

*

"I think the bathroom looks great." Sara stands wrapped in a towel, looking over the work we did today. The walls are a fresh pale yellow, and the crown molding stands out with its new white coat. She's shower clean and smells so good.

"I agree," I say, grabbing her towel from the back.

"Cash," she says in shock, turning around and covering her breasts.

"Like I haven't seen everything you have," I tell her.

"It's a natural reaction." She shrugs. I pull my bottom lip into my mouth and look her over. "For someone who has seen everything I have, you sure don't act like it," she says, giving me a small smile.

"You're beautiful," I tell her as I walk closer to her. She swallows my compliment and licks her lips. I reach up and run a finger over her belly and grab her waist, pulling her flush against me. I lean down and move her wet hair from her neck and breathe in deep. She smells like a field of lavender and honeysuckles. I taste her skin and move her so she is up against the hallway wall. Running my hand down the side of her thigh, I lift her leg and pull it around my waist. I'm fully dressed, and she stands naked. I grab her ass and suck on her neck.

Moving her head to the side, she gives me better access, and I lift her other leg, taking her feet away from the floor and surrounding myself with all of her. Her smell, her hair, her soft skin, her crazy mind, and her heart are pressed against mine. I take her to our room and lay her down. Honeysuckle love kisses my mouth and makes my heart beat faster. She grabs my T-shirt, and I help her remove it so our skin can touch. My jeans go next, and once I sink inside her, she moans into my mouth and I bite her bottom lip. I love her on the outside, like I love her on the inside. Deep and hard, rough and soft. Life-changing and earth-shattering. She's everything, and I tell her over and over.

"Never let me go."

"Not possible," she breathes.

"Promise," I urge her because I'm desperate to hear it.

"Promise, promise," she says.

*

Sara

I tap my nails against the bar top as Banner walks over.

"Hey, Sara, what can I get you?"

"I'd like a beer, please, while I wait for Maci and Leigh."

"Coming up."

I look back at the empty dance floor. It's quiet, but it's early. Banner slides me my beer, and I see the girls walk in the door.

"Hey," I say, standing up.

"Tell Maci she looks good," Leigh says with pursed lips. "She keeps saying she thinks her butt looks big in those jeans, and I think it looks just right."

"Let me see," I say. Maci turns around and shows me. "You look fine to me."

"But these jeans are so tight, I feel like you can see my cellulite," she says, and I see her dart her eyes over at Banner.

"What cellulite?" Leigh asks, sliding onto a barstool and signaling for Banner. "I've seen you in a bathing suit. You have none."

"You must have not looked good enough because I have some," she whispers harshly.

"Why are you whispering?" Leigh asks and looks at me, like *has Maci gone nuts?*

"Banner, I'd like a beer, please," Maci says, ignoring Leigh.

"Me, too," Leigh says quickly.

"Coming up, ladies."

"So, how are things?" I ask Maci.

"Things are okay," she lies. Banner puts two beers on the bar, which Maci gladly takes after she gives him a small smile.

"Cut the shit," Leigh says after taking a sip of hers. "This is us. If you're hurting, tell us. If you're sad, we're the girls you can cry in front of. The girls who don't give a crap about your makeup running or how your face looks when you ugly cry. If you're mad, we'll go smash some shit and get some frustration out. But don't play like this is okay, like this was just a bad breakup in high school and the guy won't give you back the nude pics you gave him."

Maci sighs. "Okay," she says. "Banner, pour us some shots." He does, and Maci tosses hers back and slams the shot glass down for a refill, which Banner obliges with a sly grin. She wipes her mouth and looks down at the bar, chewing on her bottom lip. "I'm sad," she says, looking back up. She looks past me, though obviously looking to see if Banner has walked off. He has. "Every day," she continues. "It's hard for me to climb out of bed. It's hard for me to find the care to brush my teeth. My heart hurts, as though it's literally been torn from my chest and slammed back in." She rubs her face and grabs her beer. "He broke me. He was my world, and he took advantage of my love and my trust and he broke them all." Heartache wipes a stray tear from her cheek and looks over at us. "Some nights I pray for the sun not to shine."

"I know exactly how you feel," I tell her. "I feel like this for no reason. A lot more than I'd like to admit."

"What do you do about it?"

I smirk. "My scars are on the outside, Maci."

Her face sobers, and she looks down. "I'm sorry, Sara. That was a stupid question."

"No, it wasn't. You're my friends. Like Leigh says, there's no point in tiptoeing around the lion. He'll know you're there. Might as well face him and get it over with. I was sad. I didn't want to be sad anymore. I didn't want to hurt anymore, so I made a decision."

"My mom killed herself," Leigh says. Maci and I look over at her. She looks at her drink. "I walked into her bathroom when I was a kid, and she was lying on the floor with her wrist pouring blood. If I had been older, maybe I could have saved her. But I wasn't." She looks up at me. "I'm sorry, Sara, but I can only think that's a selfish thing to do."

“I can see how you would think that as a person viewing it from the outside,” I say as Banner pours us another round of shots, “but depression is a disease only the depressed understand, and even then there are so many questions that just have no answers.”

*

Maci dances freely on the open dance floor, laughing and running her hands through her hair. Bright red skates over her pretty pale skin, and she smiles like she hasn’t in weeks. Leigh joins her when she walks out of the restroom, and then I get called over. Music flows through our ears, and alcohol swims through our veins. The night has been long, but like all nights with good friends, it hasn’t been long enough. I love these girls like family, and they give me just one more reason to keep going even when it’s hard.

*

I prop my feet up onto Leigh’s lap, and Maci pulls a chair over and puts her legs up, too. She’s giggly drunk, and Leigh clutches a glass of beer.

“I met Mark when I was in the seventh grade,” Leigh tells us. “I’ve never been with anyone but him.”

“I’ve only been with Cash.”

"And I've only been with Lucas."

"Don't you think we missed out?" Leigh asks.

"On what?" I say.

"On experimenting. I mean, one man for the rest of your life. There are so many men out there." She laughs.

"None that I want." I pick up my beer and have a taste.

"That's because Cash is insanely gorgeous and treats you like a queen."

"We have our rough days just like everyone else."

"What do you argue over? Who is being nicer?" Maci laughs.

"Come on, guys," I say with an eye roll. "Cash and I have been through a lot. I'm usually the problem, but he has his days where he has had enough and he'll tell me. My mood swings are unpredictable. Sometimes I'm great, but when I'm not, he has to deal with it and that can be rough on a person. So no, we don't argue about dirty clothes or the fact the floor hasn't been swept, because those things aren't important."

"That's true. They aren't," Leigh says. "Sometimes I just feel trapped."

"With Mark?" I ask.

"No, I love Mark, and honestly, if I had the chance to experiment, I know I couldn't do it. Mark makes me happy when he isn't pissing me off." She winks. "I guess what I mean is, this town is so small. There's a great big world out there. One I haven't seen any of. He wants to stay stuck in this place and have babies and a white picket fence. I'd be happy with that eventually, but first I want to see the world. Enjoy us."

"Tell him that then."

"Girl, I tell him all the time," Leigh says to Maci.

"Well, you aren't telling him right. If I know Mark, and I do, I know he loves you and would do anything to make you happy. So, you need to sit him down and tell him what you really want," Maci says, taking a sip from her beer.

Leigh sighs. "You're right. I do tell him I want to move, but I've never really told him my dreams about traveling. Maybe I will."

"What about you, Sara? Any big dreams in that head of yours?" Leigh asks me. I look down at my bottle. The lime in it fizzes, and I take a sip.

"I just want to live a full life, happy with the man I love. In a small town just like this, with good friends like you two," I say, looking up. "If you do go traveling, make sure you come back because I'll miss you."

"Me, too," Maci says. "It's not easy finding good friends like you two."

"I'll drink to that." Leigh smiles, and we clink our glasses together.

"Here's to good drinks, small towns, and the best of friends a girl could ask for," Maci toasts.

Chapter Fifteen
Sara

Colder than a few weeks ago wind blows across my face as the changing leaves get swept from one side of the road to the other. Tingles run up the back of my calves, and icy hot heat spreads throughout my lungs. I take in air through my mouth and breathe it out my nose. Sweat trickles down the center of my spine, and my thighs burn. I'm running as fast as my body will allow, chasing away bad thoughts and shifty mood swings. Today has been tough, and the walls are closing in on me. I've gone from one panic attack to another for no reason at all.

My new running shoes I bought online have soft gel bubbles at the bottom, and it's like I'm floating over the pavement. My new sports bra is filled with sweat, and my new tank top that reads *Mind Over Matter* makes me feel like a real runner and not just a girl trying to get out of her own head for a while. My therapist told me to start exercising, says it will help. So I went a little crazy and bought a bunch of stuff online. I've hidden it from Cash, which is pointless since he'll know once the credit card bill comes in. I see our driveway up ahead and run faster, until my lungs feel like they are going to explode and my leg muscles tighten.

I fall on my back, landing on the crunchy leaves and dying grass. Sweat drips down the side of my face, and I stare up at the clear blue sky. White puffy clouds move fast, and my chest does the same as my breathing tries to level. I put my hand over my stomach and wipe the sweat from my brow, thinking maybe I need to rake these leaves I'm lying on. I sit up and untie my shoes, removing them and my socks. I wiggle my toes free and stand up to walk inside. The house feels stuffy, and I drop my shoes and socks and go around opening all the windows, letting the fall breeze move in from the field. I lift my tank top over my head and drape it over my shoulder. The leaves can wait.

Taking off my running shorts and sports bra, I step into the cool shower and let the water remove the sweat from my body. It feels like heaven as I sigh and run my hands over my hair. I shut my eyes and concentrate on the water falling onto my shoulders and running down my stomach. I blink my eyes open when I hear the curtain move. "Fucking hell, Cash." I put my hand over my chest and shake my head.

"Sorry, I needed a quick shower." He smiles at me, and I seriously think my heart may pound out of my chest.

"Well, you couldn't have waited?" I ask as I blink the water out of my eyes. "What the hell is all over you?" I reach up and touch the side of his face.

"Mud," he says, moving me out of the way.

"Mud?"

"Yeah. Shit, this water is cold." He adjusts the knobs, leans his head back, and rinses off the dried-up mud.

"I went for a run."

He opens his eyes. "So, you're actually listening to Dannie?"

"Hey, I listen to Dannie. I have a journal." The water below us turns brown and orange, and I move back. "Where were you to get mud on you?"

"Mark and I kind of went off-roading this morning."

"Kind of?" I ask.

He smiles and reaches behind me for the shampoo. "Maybe, not kind of." He kisses my nose and opens the bottle. I watch him squirt some onto the palm of his hand before he gives it back to me, and I do the same.

"I thought you were helping him chop firewood?"

"I was and then we hopped on his four wheelers." He's all smiles and in a happy mood. He rinses his head and bathes off quickly before he hops out.

"Well, I'm glad you had fun."

"Me, too," he says before I hear the door shut. I roll my eyes, but can't help but smile. He needs to have more fun and act his age. He's only in his late twenties, but you'd think he was older.

You make him older.

I rinse off, too, and get out, trying to ignore the thoughts of how I make Cash's life hard.

*

Cash

Embers of fire drift upward into the night sky, dancing around each other until they burn out completely. I watch the stars with a cold beer in my hand and a tipsy Mark beside me. He's strumming a tune he only knows on the guitar, and I hear Sara, Maci, and Leigh laughing inside. Leigh walks out first with a bottle of something.

"Baby," she calls out.

Mark stops playing and looks her way. "Yeah?"

"Tell these girls how I got up on stage that one time when I turned twenty-one and almost chugged a whole bottle of tequila in one gulp." She sways a tad, and I'm guessing she doesn't need what's inside that bottle.

"You did."

"But tell them," she says again.

"She did!" he yells.

She nods her head and opens the door. "Thanks," she says. "See, I told you two I did it." I hear her say before the door shuts again.

"She really did that?" I ask.

"Yep, she spent the whole night with her face in the toilet, too."

I laugh and take a swig of my beer. Mark puts the guitar down and stands up. He kicks a log deeper into the fire pit before he sits back down and grabs a beer from the cooler. "So, how's she doing, man?" he asks me as he pops the top.

I look over at him and then back down at the fire. "She's good," I say, but I don't tell him about two nights ago when she broke a whole rack of dishes because her mood went from happy to pissed-the-fuck-off in two seconds. I don't tell him about the credit card bills and how she has clothes with tags still on them. I keep my mouth shut about the tears she cries for no reason and how her meds make her sleepy and she keeps going to her shrink because sometimes she isn't sure about life. Hell, we hardly talk about it between the two of us, so there's no reason for me to talk about it with him. "Yeah, man, she's doing good." I swallow my lie with cold beer and lean back in my chair.

Lying is easy when you're protecting the person you love. You don't want anyone to judge them harshly, so you don't give them any reason to. You can because it's your love, but nobody else better fucking do it, so you lie. You lie to keep them happy; you lie to keep yourself believing everything is okay—that your life is normal. That it's fine your wife sometimes would rather stay in the dark than see the sunshine. You talk yourself up and you make yourself believe that she'll be all right, and if she isn't, you'll do everything in your power to make her be.

"Glad to hear that, man."

I nod and look toward the house of laughing females. The screen door opens, and out they walk. Leigh holds on to that same bottle, while Sara jogs down the steps and straight to me. She sits on my lap and links her fingers behind my neck.

"What are you two doing out here?" she asks me.

"This and that." I grin.

"This and that," she counters. I bounce my knee so she bounces, too. She smiles and looks up at the sky. "It's a perfect night."

"It is," I agree, looking up just as a star shoots across the sky.

"Did you see that?" Sara asks, wide-eyed.

"I did."

"Make a wish, baby," she tells me as she closes her eyes. I close mine, too, and wish for more perfect days just like this one.

"Did you wish?" she asks.

"Yes."

"What did you wish for?"

"I can't tell you."

She grins. "You're no fun, Cash Williams."

"If I tell you, it won't come true."

"Did you wish for babies?" she asks me quietly. I look over her pretty face. It's slightly flushed from drinking, and her hair falls carelessly around it.

"Did *you*?" I ask.

"Maybe." She shrugs.

"We can work on that, you know? All you have to do is stop taking your birth control."

"I know." She smiles, and then her face turns serious as though she had a bad thought.

"I'm getting tired," she says, sliding off my lap. "I'm going to call it a night, guys." She walks away and into the house as the girls tell her bye. Leigh looks over at me with a concerned expression. I look away.

"She's had a long day," I say. Like I said, lying for the people you love is easy, and soon you become so good at it you don't know what the truth is anymore. Sara hasn't had a long day; she slept most of it away and actually didn't get up until I told her everyone was coming over, and I only did that to get her out of bed. She can't be tired, or maybe she can. Who really knows?

*

I walk into the house after I put the fire out and everyone leaves. Sara sits at the kitchen counter with a cup of coffee in her hand.

"Why did you do that?" she asks me.

"Do what?" I question as I lean against the doorway.

"Invite everyone over, knowing I was tired today."

"You slept all day, Sara. How in the hell can you be tired still?" I push off the doorframe and walk around the countertop.

“You don’t know what I am or how I feel, Cash, so stop acting like you do.”

“I’m just saying you slept all day. There is no way a person can still be tired if they slept for fourteen hours.”

“I can,” she says. “I could sleep for a week and probably still be tired.”

“Well, then we need to get your medicine fixed.”

“Fuck my medicine. I’m sick to death of taking that shit. I’m tired of getting it changed all the damn time. Nothing helps. Nothing helps with these shifty feelings I have.” She slides off the stool and dumps her coffee into the sink. “I’m never going to feel normal, and I don’t want to bring a kid into this world and risk them feeling like I do. I can’t put that on anyone else.”

“You’re the one talking about having babies, Sara. I never mentioned it.” She doesn’t say anything back, but her eyes fill with tears.

“I hate myself.”

“Don’t say that.”

“It’s true. I hate myself. I hate everything. I hate this stupid house. I hate this stupid kitchen. I hate this coffee mug.” She picks it up and smashes it onto the floor. “I hate you!” she screams, walking over broken glass and running out of here. The sting in my chest is the only thing she leaves. That and the small drops of blood on the floor.

*

I walk out onto the porch and sit down, running my hands over my face and looking out. The moonlight casts a glow on the road, and smoke still rises from the fire pit in the yard. I know Sara doesn't hate me, but damn, if those words coming from her mouth don't hurt. I hear the screen door open, and I turn to see her. She leans against it and puts her hands behind her back.

"Cash, I'm so sorry," she says with tears in her eyes, and I know she is.

"Come here, baby," I say, holding out my hand. She takes it eagerly, and I pull her onto my lap. She wraps her arm around my neck, and I put my face in her hair and breathe her in. She smells like fire and broken promises. One day she is going to hate herself too much, and that'll be the end of everything. I fear that day so terribly it makes my hands tremble. She cries, and I breathe. She hurts, and I do, too. Our hearts beat the same rhythm, and our souls are made from the same star, but her mind fights it and it ruins us both.

"I love you," I tell her. "I'll love you even when we are nothing but a faded memory."

"Promise me," she says.

"Promise, promise, baby."

Chapter Sixteen
Sara

I flip through the pages of my journal, skimming over words I've written throughout the past few months. Happy days, sad days, crazy days, and days filled with all emotions inside a different hour. I'm all over the place, and I toss the book aside and open the cap on my medicine bottle. Two pills fall out onto my hand, and I throw them back, chasing them with a glass of water from my nightstand.

"Today is going to be a good day, Sara." I talk myself up and take a deep breath before I stand, wincing as soon as I do because I cut my foot pretty bad from stepping over the broken mug. Sighing, I pull a sweater over my head. You can feel the cold wind coming in from the old windows. The house holds a constant chill, and they say we may get snow today. We shall see.

I walk out of the bedroom and down the stairs. Cash sits on the couch with a foot propped up on the coffee table. I walk over and sit down beside him. He puts his arm around me, and I lift my foot and hug my knee. I take medicine that doesn't work, and I'll be so tired in a little while, I'll probably fall asleep right here. That is, if Cash lets me.

"Your mom called while you were getting dressed."

"Oh, yeah?" I ask.

"Yep."

"I'll call her later."

"Up to you." He shrugs.

"How long has it been now?" I ask.

"Since when?"

"Since you've spoken to your parents."

"A while." He looks down.

"You should call them."

"Why?"

"Because life's too short. Because I know you miss them."

"They didn't support me, Sara. They didn't support us."

"I know that, but people mess up."

"Yeah, but who doesn't show up to their son's wedding?"

"I'm sure they regret it."

"Maybe so." He sighs and pulls me closer. I feel his lips on my forehead, and I snuggle up to him. My eyes look out the window in our living room, and I jump up.

"Baby, it's snowing." I move away from him and walk to the door. Pulling it open, I step out onto the front porch. A smile spreads across my face. I hear Cash walk up behind me.

"They're saying we may get a good bit. You want to head to the store now and pick up some things and some more of your smell-good candles in case the lights go out?"

"Yeah, let me go put my shoes on." I tuck a stray curl behind my ear and turn around. Cash leans against the front door. His arms are crossed over his chest, and his dark hair is getting long. His beard shields his face, but it's not overpowering. My husband is so good-looking.

"What are you staring at, baby?"

"You." I smile and walk up to him. He licks his lips before I softly plant mine onto his. It's quick, and I pull away. "I love you. I don't deserve you, but I love you with my whole heart," I tell pure love.

"I deserve you, though, and I love you with my whole life." He wraps me in a hug, and I breathe in his scent. It's fresh air and a stream of springtime water flowing down a mountaintop. It's manly. It's Cash.

“Let’s go to the store before the roads get too bad,” he says, and we walk inside so I can grab my shoes.

*

The snow comes down in sheets as we head to town. With no heat in Old Blue, it’s freezing. I sit in the middle so I can keep warm beside Cash. Our breaths blow smoke, and I wish he had driven the police truck home Friday evening. We turn into town and come to a stop at the red light. I see white smoke bellowing out of the tailpipe in the side mirror as Mark walks across the street. Cash rolls his window down. “Hey, man, you need me to come help you with some more firewood?” Cash asks.

“Yeah, but it can wait. Come on by the house, though, and I’ll send you home with some for helping me the other day.” Mark puts his hands into his pockets. “They say it’s going to get really bad later tonight.”

“That’s what I heard. I’ll make my way over there after we get finished here.”

“Sounds good. I get off in about twenty minutes.”

Cash nods before Mark hurries across the road. We park the truck, and Cash gives me a quick kiss before we get out. His lips are cold, and I know mine are, too.

"We have to get that heater fixed," I say.

"We will." He grabs my icy fingers and pulls the door open. I instantly thaw out from the warmness inside the store.

"So, what should we get?" Cash asks as we scan the aisles.

"Junk food and meat." I grin.

"That's my wife." He winks.

After we clean the shelves in the candy aisle, we walk over to the meat and grab a few steaks and some other things to put into our freezer. We walk to the checkout line, and I look over the magazines. Someone is having a baby with this person and someone is adopting two kids from another country. Twelve million dollar divorce for these two people. Geez, I thought I had problems.

"I'm sorry, sir, but your card has been declined."

I look up at the cashier.

"Here, try this one." Cash hands her another card, and I bite my bottom lip, praying it goes through. Shit, did I use that one recently? I exhale air I didn't know I was holding when the receipt prints and she hands it to Cash. I grab some bags and follow him out. I can see from the tension in his shoulders, he is pissed. He opens my door for me to get in, but he doesn't look at me.

“Cash.”

“Just get in, Sara.”

I do and he shuts the door. Once he’s inside, he sits still, holding his hands over the steering wheel. He looks out the front windshield, and I look down at his jaw as it ticks.

“Is it going to come down to me hiding my wallet from you?” he finally says.

“Cash…I.”

“No, Sara. I don’t want to hear you’re sorry. I want to know. Is this the kind of relationship you want to have? Where we have to hide things from each other?” He glances over at me, and I look away. “Because I’ll do it. I’ll fucking hide every piece of money we own or make if it keeps us from having credit cards being denied.”

“Oh, you’re going to get upset at me? What about the motorcycle you bought, Cash? You didn’t talk to me about it. You just bought it, and I didn’t flip out on you.”

“I thought it would make you happy, baby. Plus, that was before redoing the house drained us.”

I sigh and look out the window. “Can you just take me home, please?” I see him shake his head before he starts the truck. The ride back is quiet, and once we make it home, we carry the bags inside.

"I'm heading over to Mark's for a bit. I'll be back in a little while." He grabs his keys and looks back at me. "Okay?" he asks.

"Okay."

He walks out, and I close my eyes and grip the countertop behind me when the door shuts. I decide to take a nap. The covers welcome me, and the darkness in my room comforts my mind and mood. Sometime later sleep takes over.

*

Cash

I lift my arm and quickly bring it back down onto the piece of wood in front of me. Snow falls, and it's freezing here. Mark told me not to worry about cutting up any more, but I need to get this anger out. I'm pissed. I'm pissed off at my wife. I'm pissed off at myself. I should have been more careful. I should have hidden our credit cards from her. But that pisses me off more because I shouldn't have to hide shit from her. She is my wife. My partner.

Lifting my arm again, I slam down hard onto the firewood. It splits one piece, becoming two halves, separating and falling away from each other. I step back and look at the two splintered pieces of oak. Sara's disorder is the ax, and we are the logs. I blink my eyes and look around at the white snow that covers the ground. I feel how cold it is and see the smoke coming from my mouth. I toss the ax away from me. Fuck that ax.

*

Sara

I jump awake and look over at the clock. It's two in the morning, and I still feel tired. Cash sleeps soundly beside me, and I toss the covers off and rake a hand through my hair. Looking out, I see the glow of the moonlight shining against the night sky. The frosty windows creak, and a chill runs over my arms as the wind howls outside. I touch my toes to the hardwood. I see the deep hole my mind wants to crawl into, and every part of me is fighting to stay out of it. The bottom of my foot touches the floor, and I stand up and walk to the closet. I slip my boots on and a coat over my nightgown. A scarf mindlessly goes around my neck, and without much thought, I walk down the stairs and out the front door.

*

Cash

My eyes blink open, and I run a hand over my face. I reach over and feel that the bed is empty. Looking to the clock, I see it's almost three in the morning. "Sara."

She doesn't answer, and I get up. After I check the bathroom and see she isn't there, I run down the stairs and look in the kitchen. "Sara," I call out into the house. Panic is a sudden form of fear or anxiety, but this in my chest is worse when I see the door is unlocked. I slip my boots on and grab my coat. Zipping it up, I open the door and heavy snow and painfully cold wind greet me. "Sara!" I look out into the yard. It's dark, so I run back inside and grab my flashlight. I turn it on and point it to the ground, searching for her tracks. Moving it back and forth, I see them and quickly follow. My feet move as quickly as they can, but it's hard to see with the snow blowing around me. My pajamas are soaked at the bottom, and the wetness is crawling up my legs, making my teeth chatter. I point the flashlight toward the old tree in the field and see her.

She's walking under it where the snow isn't so thick. My heart falls at the sight of her out here. The snow blows around her. Her arms are crossed, and she mindlessly wanders. What can she be thinking? What is going on in her mind? I take off running toward her. I run as fast as I can until I'm close enough to scoop her up into my arms. "Baby."

She stills in my arms, and her body shakes from tears I don't have to see to know are falling. I turn her around and look at her face. Her nose and cheeks are rosy red. I cradle her against my chest and walk back, trying to keep her warm and not fall at the same time. Once I'm at the door, I kick it open and put her down on the couch.

Quickly, I take some logs and toss them into the fireplace. Lighting it as fast as I can, I grab some pillows off the couch and put them in front of it. Taking my coat off, I walk over to a spaced-out Sara and remove her boots and then her coat. She looks ahead, not seeming to be focused on anything, but everything at once. I can tell her mind is racing, and she can't keep up with its speed. "Come down here, baby. I've got to get you warm." She lets me pull her down to the floor, and I sit behind her on the pillows, wrapping my arms around her waist and holding her tight. I kiss the top of her hair and rest my chin on her head as I look at the flames in the fireplace. The wood crackles, and my heart won't stop pounding.

"I'm a burning house," she murmurs.

"What, Sara?" I ask.

"I'm a burning house, and you're stuck inside. Soon I won't be anything but ash, and I'm going to take you right down with me," she cries. This time I can't find the words to comfort her

because they are stuck in my throat along with tears
I won't let fall.

Chapter Seventeen
Cash

"I can't watch her. I have to go to work. Can you please come out?"

"Of course," Debbie says. "I'll be there tomorrow."

"Thanks." I hang up the phone and look out the window. Snow continues to fall, but it's not the storm outside I'm worried about. It's the one inside my wife's head. Sara has gone into a deep depression. She's sleeping soundlessly on the couch. I won't take my eyes off of her unless someone else's are on her. The power went out last night but came back on this morning. The fire has kept the living room warm, but every other part of the house is playing catch-up. I walk over to the coffeepot and pour myself a cup.

Surprisingly, Sara woke up to take her medication earlier, but she immediately went back to sleep. Taking a sip of my coffee, I daydream out the window. I hear a car pull up outside, so I put the cup down and walk to the front door. I slide one hand into my pocket and open the door with the other. Chilly wind blows in from outside, and I place my other hand in to keep warm.

"Hey." Leigh is in a good mood, but her best friend isn't.

"She's sleeping, Leigh. We had a rough night," I tell this girl because she knows her friend's story.

"Oh, well darn. Now that the snow has lightened up some, I wanted to see if she wanted to get out of the house."

"Yeah, today isn't a good day. I'll tell her you came by, though," I say, shaking my arms a tad to try to keep warm.

"Okay, I'll call later." She's disappointed and worried when she gets back into the car, and as she drives away, I think that's exactly how I feel. Disappointed and worried. After Sara tried to kill herself a year ago, I thought she was getting better. I thought maybe we wouldn't have to go through this again. Even though Dannie, her therapist, told me this was just part of my wife's syndrome. She will get sad, she will get mad, and she will be indifferent. She will have days where you can't keep up. Days she goes from one emotion to the other. She may go on spending binges or get obsessively wrapped up in something to the point it becomes unhealthy. I have to watch the signs. The signs. Which fucking signs? There are so many. I can't keep up.

I shut the door and walk over to the stack of firewood. Grabbing a log, I toss it into the fire and rest my arm on the mantel as sparks fly up. Mindlessly, I watch the wood burn. Sara mumbles, and I cast my eyes over to her.

"Baby, how are you feeling?" I ask. She doesn't respond, so I let her be and walk back into the kitchen. I sit down with my coffee and put my face into my hands. I pray for my wife, I pray for myself, and I pray for my heart because it's a beat away from crumbling.

*

Sara

I roll over in our bed and see that I'm the only one in it. "Cash," I call out. My voice is raspy from sleeping so much, and my head hurts. "Cash," I say again. The door to our bedroom opens, and I blink from the light coming in from the hallway. "Mama?" I ask, sitting up.

"Yes, baby girl." She walks in and sits down on the bed.

"Why are you here? Where's Cash?"

"He had to go to work. He asked me to come stay with you."

I don't say anything, because what's the point? They do what they want anyway.

"Are you hungry? You've been asleep for a while now."

"I could eat a little." I move my hair away from my face and take the covers off of me.

"You going to come down and eat?" she asks me.

"Yeah."

"Can I get you some clothes?"

"No, I'll wear what I have on," I say, looking down at my nightgown.

"But it's the middle of the day, Sara. Don't you think you should get dressed? Let's take down these dark blankets from the windows."

I put my feet down, stand up, and walk into the bathroom. I shut the door, ignoring her. I don't want to put any damn clothes on. I want to wear this, and I like my dark blankets. I roll my eyes when I hear her mumbling as she walks out of the room. Why did Cash call her? I turn the faucet on and cup my hands underneath the water. I put my face down and hold my breath as the water presses against my skin. It feels good. I lean up and grab a towel, wiping the water off and looking at myself in the mirror. Dark circles are under my eyes, and my hair is wild. Shrugging, I grab my toothbrush.

*

"You can't eat any more than that?" Mama asks me as disapproval shows on her face.

"I'm full." I get up and rake the rest into the trashcan.

"Sara, you hardly ate a thing." She wipes the countertop, and I inhale a deep breath.

"I ate what I wanted, Mama."

"How are you to gain any weight if you eat like a bird?"

"Who said I wanted to gain any weight?"

"Well, no one did, but you do. You are far too skinny."

I look down at my body. "I think I look fine."

"You look as though you don't eat enough. Does Cash not keep food in this house?"

"Don't start."

"All you have are junk food and frozen meat in this kitchen. You need some vegetables and fruits."

"Mama, I said not to start."

"I'm just saying, Sara. A person…"

I throw my plate down onto the floor, and it shatters. Glass slides across the floor.

"I said not to fucking start. I don't want to hear your bullshit judgments. This is my house, Cash is my husband, and we take care of each other just fine. We don't need you coming in here and trying to change things."

Mama stands there with a hand over her mouth. I shake my head and walk over to the broom.

"Sara, you need to go see the doctor. This is getting out of hand."

I grip the broom handle and bite my tongue. Where the hell is my husband? I'm going to kick his ass for asking her to come here.

*

Cash

"Thanks for bringing the firewood by, Cash," Maci says.

"It's not a problem."

"How's Sara feeling today? Leigh said she came by yesterday, and she wasn't feeling great."

"Yeah, she's okay. Her mom is visiting."

“Oh, well, I hope that’s going all right.” Maci makes a face. I laugh.

“Yeah, me, too. How’ve you been doing?”

“I’m okay. I take it one day at a time.”

“Heard anything from Lucas?”

“He writes.”

I wait for her to continue, but she doesn’t and I don’t want to pry.

“Okay, well, we’ll see you later then.”

“Thanks again.”

*

I stop by the Kingsley’s house to give them some firewood, but really I’m just checking to see if they are getting along. Joe walks out to meet me.

“Afternoon, deputy.”

“Joe.” I nod. “You guys get along okay during the storm?”

“Yep, saw a big tree fall in the backyard, and the lights went out for a bit, but we’re good.”

“Glad to hear it. I brought you two some firewood.”

"Thanks. We're running low, and my heater is working on overdrive." He walks on down to help me unload the wood.

"How's Elizabeth?"

"She's taking a nap right now. I don't know how, though. She's had five cups of coffee."

"You got her a new pot?" I ask.

"Yep." He grins.

*

Walking into the bar, I see Drew sitting, babysitting a beer. His chief's hat sits on the bar top. I make my way over and have a seat, too.

"How are the Kingsleys doing?" he asks me.

"Fine. They had a tree fall in the backyard. Figured once the snow thaws, we could go over and help Joe cut it."

"Yeah, I'll see if Guzman will help." He takes a sip of his beer and makes an *ahh* sound. "Nothing like a cold one after a long day's work."

"True story," I agree as I lift my finger for Banner to get me one. He nods my way.

"Did you stop by the office before you got here?" the chief asks me.

"Yeah, Anne said she was going ahead and closing up, said she has some grocery shopping to do for Thanksgiving."

"That's what I was wondering. She goes all out on these holidays. We still got a few weeks, and she's stocking our freezer up."

"Sara is all about Christmas. I imagine the house will be filled with decorations."

"It's good to be into something," Drew says. "How's she doing anyway?"

I sigh. "Some days are better than others. Her mom is visiting right now."

"Oh, you get along good with her family?"

"For the most part. Her dad is better than her mom."

"Yeah," he says. "Anne's dad never did like me much. He said I was trouble, and his girl didn't need to be around me." Drew laughs. "I was into everything in my younger years. I swear, if you would have told me I'd grow up to be the chief of police, I would have laughed in your face and called you a fool."

"You were a troublemaker?" I ask, not believing him.

"Shoot yeah, I didn't believe in following the rules."

I laugh and grab my beer that Banner put on the bar.

"What about you?" the chief asks me.

"I was an okay kid. My dad was the sheriff, so I didn't get into trouble much."

"Ahh, the sheriff's kid is usually the worst they say."

"I think that's the preacher's kid," I say, taking a swig from my bottle. He laughs.

"You're probably right. Well, I think I better be getting to the house, son. Anne will need help unloading those groceries. You and Sara got any plans for Turkey Day?" he asks, standing up and placing his hat on his head.

"Figured her mom will cook or something."

He nods and tosses some bills onto the bar. "Well if that doesn't pan out, you know you're more than welcome at ours."

"'Preciate that," I say. He pats my shoulder and tilts his hat toward Banner before walking out.

*

"I can't deal with her anymore," Sara says in a harsh whisper. She dumps clean clothes onto the bed and drops the basket onto the floor. "I called

Dannie today. I have an appointment tomorrow, so there is no need in me having a babysitter here."

"You called Dannie?" I ask.

"Yes," she says, looking over at me. She puts down the shirt in her hand and rubs her face after she sits on the bed. Her hair is piled on top of her head, and she wears a tank top and wrap with loose fitted jeans. She got dressed, so that's a plus.

"These holes I get in take a lot out of me. This medicine isn't working once again. I'm sick to death with feeling like this. So yeah, I called Dannie. I guess I need to talk it out, but my mom being here doesn't help a damn thing. I love the woman, but she drives me crazy, baby." She looks over at me and shakes her head. "How did I live with her for so long?"

I laugh. "I wonder that, too."

She smiles, and it's the first one I've seen in days, so I smile back. She sighs and falls back onto the bed, throwing her arms above her head. Her eyes blink, and I watch her. She looks over at me and holds her arms up, like *come here*. So I do. I climb on top of her, holding my weight off of her small body. She looks into my eyes and wraps her arms around my neck. "How was your day?" she asks me, looking from my eyes to my lips.

"Better now." I lean down and take her bottom lip between my teeth. She closes her eyes as my tongue touches hers, and she pulls me down closer. There's a knock on the door. Opening her eyes, love sighs and then rolls her eyes. I laugh lightly.

"My mom is a cock blocker," Sara says, and I burst out laughing as I climb off of her and walk to the door.

"Wondering what you two would like for supper? I've found some potatoes that aren't rotten and you have chicken in the freezer."

I look back when Sara speaks. "Mama, we have more than chicken, but anyway, you don't need to cook us supper. We can just go grab something, and you can head on home to Daddy."

"You could use a home-cooked meal."

My wife links her arm with her mom's after she walks past me. "I think I'll be okay," she says, forcing her mom to walk with her because their arms are joined. I follow them down the hall with a smile on my face. Sara is kicking Debbie out, but in the nicest way. We walk down the stairs with Debbie telling Sara she needs to eat more and eat healthier. Sara just nods. Debbie even suggests her daughter needs to go grocery shopping more. She looks back at me and says, "You need to take better care of Sara and make sure she takes her meds every day. This house could use some cleaning, too. If you want, I can help you."

Sara grabs her mom's purse from the table behind the couch as we walk past it. I walk ahead and open the front door. "I love you, Mama. As always, thank you for coming."

Sara kisses Debbie's cheek and unlinks their arms before she hands Chatty Cathy her purse.

"Just take care of yourself," Debbie says to her child.

"Always, Mama."

Debbie puts her purse strap over her shoulder and looks to me. "Call me if you need anything."

"Will do, Debbie," I say, still holding the door open. "Have a safe trip home." Debbie walks out.

"Send my love to Daddy," Sara calls out, giving her mom one last wave before we shut the door. "Holy shit," Sara tells me with wide eyes. "That woman will make you want to pull your damn hair out." She walks into the kitchen and puts the chicken back into the freezer. "Want a burger?" she asks me, and I grin.

"Sounds good."

Chapter Eighteen
Cash

I look over at the clock. It's two in the morning. Baby isn't in the bed, and I'm not surprised. She's on a mission. Thanksgiving is being held at our place, and she hasn't stopped going since she decided to host it. I roll over and grab her pillow. Breathing in, I smell her scent, and sometime later, I fall back asleep.

*

"Everything looks great, Sara." I pick up a loose piece of turkey from the bottom of the pan and pop it into my mouth.

"Cash, get your hands out of that!" My wife slaps my arm and moves around me to cover the turkey. "Is it moist enough?" She blows a piece of stray hair out of her face and wipes her brow with the back of her hand.

"It's delicious. Don't worry. No one is expecting it to be perfect. It's your first time hosting."

"You mean, it's my first time cooking like this."

"Well…yeah, that, too." I wink and give her a kiss on the cheek. She smells like cooking and clean linen.

"And who's worrying?" She grins and grabs the boiled eggs off the stove. "I'm going to rock this dinner. I may have never cooked like this before, but I think it's all turning out pretty damn good." I narrow my eyes at her and watch as she moves around the kitchen. She's in full force. All of her energy and mind have been focused on this Thanksgiving dinner for a week now. I've tried to get her to chill out, but she tells me she's fine. She isn't fine. She's on a high, and I'm just hoping this one doesn't have a hard fall. I hear a knock on the door.

"Oh shit, whoever that is, they're early," Sara says as I wipe my hands on a dishtowel.

"Who cares? I'll entertain them while you get things ready, and if it's Leigh, maybe she can help you before you know who shows up." I walk out before she responds and open the door.

"Happy Turkey Day!" Leigh says, walking in the house. She pats my arm when she walks past me.

"She's in the kitchen," I call back to her.

"Hey, man," I say to Mark as he walks in.

"Got the game on?" he asks.

"You know it. Want a beer?"

"Yeah, thanks."

*

Sara

"I've been cooking since last night. I hope this turns out good. You know my mama will have something to say."

"So what? Let me help with something," Leigh says, tying on an apron.

"You can mash the potatoes." I take the masher out of the drawer and hand it to her. "They're over there on the counter. I've already put salt and pepper in the bowl. The butter is by the stove." I pour sugar into the sweet tea I'm making and look back toward Leigh as I pick up the wooden spoon to stir it. "So, Maci is with her parents?" I ask.

"That's what she says," Leigh replies.

"What? You don't believe her?"

"I'm grabbing Mark and me a beer," Cash says, walking into the kitchen. "What time is everyone supposed to get here?"

"In about thirty minutes," I say as he opens the fridge.

"You two want one?"

"Yes," we both say at the same time.

*

I hear the sound of everyone laughing from the living room, and I sigh. I think this is good. I think I've done well. Yeah, I've outdone myself. I untie my apron just as Mama walks into the kitchen.

"You should have put the potato salad in the fridge. No one likes hot potato salad." She grabs the bowl and puts it into the fridge.

"It's time to eat now, Mama."

"I don't know why you didn't already put it in there," she huffs, and I roll my eyes.

"Always have something to say."

"What was that?"

"Nothing," I say, picking up a bowl of peas and taking it into the dining room. The whole house is decorated, but my table looks the best. I've been putting money aside from the library, and I admit I went a little nuts on the décor purchases, but so what? It's Thanksgiving.

"Cash, will you come get the turkey?" I ask. He puts his beer down on the table and stands up. I walk back into the kitchen and grab more food.

"You're going to burn your rolls," Mama says as she takes them out of the oven. They're perfectly brown. No one is burning shit. I don't say anything to her.

"Where's the bird?" Cash walks in and smiles.

*

Cash

The food is good, and everyone tells Sara so. She nods and gives a small smile, but I can tell something is off. She shifts in her seat and looks down at her plate. Her mama is asking how much money she spent on all these decorations and food. And that's exactly what I can't stand about the woman. What's it her business? I take a bite of my food and look over at Sara when I hear a fork clink down hard on a plate. "It's none of your damn business," she snaps loudly toward her mom. Everyone stops eating and looks at Sara.

"Sara," I say, reaching my hand over at her.

"No." She snatches her hand away, and I swallow. Here it is. Here is the blow up. "This food is terrible," she says, sliding her plate away. "Everything is overcooked, isn't it, Mama?"

"I think it's great," Mark says.

"It's shit," Sara replies.

"Sara," I repeat.

"I'm sick to death of looking at it."

"You did a good job," I tell her.

"Oh, that's perfect, isn't it, Cash? Go ahead and tell everyone how good of a job I did, like I'm five." She roughly slides her chair back and tosses her napkin onto the table before she walks away. I run a hand over my face and look around. Our friends and her family sit here, all eyes on me.

"I think we should call it a day," I say. "I'm sorry."

"It's totally fine, Cash," Leigh says. "We were finished anyway. Let me help put some of this up." She turns to Debbie. "Debbie, would you mind helping me?"

"You don't have to worry about that," I say.

"It's not a problem." Leigh stands and grabs a few bowls from the table. I look over at Walter, like *why didn't you shut your wife up?*

*

"I really appreciate you helping clean things up," I say to Leigh as they start to walk out.

"I didn't mind a bit. I'm really sorry about earlier."

"Cash, please, don't be. We're your friends—next best thing to family. We understand."

"Thanks."

I shake Mark's hand and shut the door after they walk out. "She can't be on the right medications if she has mood swings this badly." Debbie enters the living room, and Walter walks behind her.

"Cash, you need to—"

"Debbie, do you ever shut up?" I ask. Her eyes go wide, and Walter doesn't say anything. "Your daughter has been in that kitchen since yesterday cooking, trying to make it perfect, because she knew you would have something to say. And you did, over and over! No, her medication doesn't work half the time. Yes, we have gone and gotten it changed. Yes, she spent a good bit of money on food and decorations. But just shut up about it!"

"Well..." Debbie says.

“Well, my ass,” I reply, opening the door. “We’ll talk soon.”

Debbie storms past me, but Walter stops. He gives me a grin, and I can’t help it, so I burst out laughing.

“See you later, my boy. Take care of our girl.”

“Yes, sir,” I reply before he walks out.

*

I walk up the stairs and into our bedroom. Sara lies sleeping. Exhaustion has finally taken over her, and I’m glad she can sleep. Maybe her high is over, and she’s had her blow up. I’m hoping that’s as bad as it gets. I walk back down and grab a beer out of the fridge before I sit down in front of the TV. I watch the game until I’m drunk and pass out on the couch. Happy fucking Thanksgiving.

Chapter Nineteen
Sara

While driving through town to go to my doctor's appointment, I see Christmas lights being hung and a big tree being pulled upright by a few men and a rope. Turning into the doctor's office, I park Old Blue and step out of the truck. It's freezing today, and snow covers the ground still from the small storm we had last night. I open the door and step inside, grateful that there is only one other person in here.

After I sign in, I grab a cup of complimentary coffee to warm my insides. I was supposed to go to the doctor after Thanksgiving, but I just couldn't get out of bed unless it was to go to work.

"Sara." My name is called, and I stand up. Tossing the coffee into the trash, I follow the nurse to the back. The hallways are lined with old photos from way back when, and the smell of new carpet hits my nose. We turn, and I see Dannie's office door is open. "She's expecting you. You can go on in."

I nod and walk into the office.

"Sara, how are you?" Dannie asks as she stands and points to the chair for me to sit.

"Good today, thanks."

"Great, so what seems to be the problem?" She sits back down in her chair, and it squeaks. She links her fingers and rests them on the desktop.

"A lot of shift in my moods lately. My meds just make me sleepy, and once again they don't seem to be working."

"Hmm… How is life going at home?"

"Well, some days are better than others. I'm a lot to handle." I kind of laugh, but Dannie doesn't.

"I went a little crazy with the credit cards and flipped out at Thanksgiving."

"Tell me all about it," Dannie says. I tell her how Cash and I argued after we left the store because of the card being denied, how I walked out of the house during a snowstorm, and how I was on a high and snapped at Thanksgiving. Saying all of this out loud makes me feel crazy. But the good thing about Dannie is, she doesn't judge.

"Well, let's see what we can do, shall we?" she says.

*

Thirty minutes later, I'm walking out with a handful of new prescriptions. Yay me. I breathe in the fresh air as I walk to Old Blue, quickly jumping inside to get out of the wind. I crank him up and head to the pharmacy to fill my bottles of sanity. Coming to a stoplight, I see Leigh walking a dog that looks like he isn't quite out of the puppy stage. With some elbow power, I roll the window down.

"Hey, dog walker!" I yell over to her. She turns my way and smiles, then quickly runs over to me before the light changes.

"Hey, yourself. What are you up to?"

"Just left the doctor."

"Everything okay?" she asks.

"Yeah, I'm good. What you got there?" I ask, looking down at the brown dog.

"This here is Bear. He's a Lab. He just showed up at the back of Banner's Bar with no collar. Sweet as ever and smart, too."

I look up when the light turns green, but there is no one behind me.

"Sit, Bear," Leigh says, and he does. She gives him a treat from her pocket, and he takes it gladly.

I smile. “He seems like a good dog. Hate he has no home.”

“You want him?” She grins as a car horn blows behind me.

“I gotta go. I’ll call you later.”

“Okay, I’ll get an answer from you later then,” she says on a wink.

“I don’t think so,” I reply, smiling as I roll the window back up and step on the gas.

*

“How did the doc go?” Maci asks as I walk into the library. Snow comes in behind me, and I take my scarf and gloves off.

“Same as always. She asked me how I was feeling. I told her some days are better than others. But I’ve been down lately, so she asked more questions and did a few tests. Now I have new medicine.”

“Sounds fun.” She lifts her brow and gives me a smirk.

“The best,” I say. “I saw Leigh walking a dog before I got here. Cute dog.”

“Watch out. She’ll be sending him home with you.”

"She tried to." I laugh as I walk around the counter and see an envelope from the state prison. I lay my gloves and scarf down and start unbuttoning my coat.

"So, you haven't said anything about Lucas in a while. You two talk or…?"

"He writes me."

"I can see that," I say, looking back down at the letter. She looks, too, and clears her throat. "You writing him back?"

She shrugs and types another book into the computer.

"Why are you being so vague?"

"I'm not."

"Yes, you are. What's the deal?"

She sighs. "The deal is, I'm confused, Sara. I love him, and I can't help it."

"He treated you like shit, Maci."

"You don't think I know that? I lived it, remember?"

I sit down on the stool and bite my lip. She rubs her forehead and looks past the computer.

"You can't help what your heart feels. I want to hate him. I really do, but it's easier said than done. I've loved that man as long as I can remember, Sara," she says, glancing over at me. "I can't just shut feelings like that off. If I could, I would."

"Okay," I say, holding up my hands. "But I don't care what he says. He doesn't love you." I point at her. "You do not treat someone you love like that, Maci. You just don't." I stand and look over at my friend who has tears in her eyes. With a heavy sigh, I look down. "I care about you, is all. Please…just be careful."

"I will. Thanks for your concern."

"Of course. I'm going to check the bucket." Walking into the restroom, I see the bucket is half full of water, so I pick it up and dump it into the sink. I can't believe she is second-guessing all of this. Lucas is a complete asshole. I know she loves him, but seriously, he held her at gunpoint. I shake my head and put the bucket back down before I walk out.

Chapter Twenty
Cash

Christmastime has always been my wife's favorite, and because it's hers, it's mine, too. I grab the decorations from out of the attic and place them in the living room.

"Let's hang some on the outside of the house first, baby."

"Really?" I ask because I know it's a damn job.

"Yes, really. It's not Christmas without lights. Come on," she says, grabbing the box of lights and setting it beside the door. She puts her coat on and turns to me as she buttons it up. "I can't seem to get the chill out of my bones in this house. You think we could sleep in the living room tonight near the fireplace?"

"Our backs will be sore as shit."

"But I'll be warm." She places her green knit hat on her head and smiles.

"You'll be warm with me beside you and blankets piled on top of us." I put my coat and gloves on before I lift the box up.

"You're no fun, Cash Williams. Pallets are the best." She opens the door, and the wind brushes against my cheeks, freezing my nose.

"Pallets were fun when we were kids, baby. Now we're old, and we have old people's backs."

"You have an old person's back. There isn't a thing wrong with mine."

"Sleep on the floor then. Tomorrow, you'll be telling me a different story about old people's backs, baby cakes."

"Baby cakes?" she says, grinning. I shrug.

"Just came out."

"Okay…baby cakes."

"Don't call me that. It doesn't sound right when you call a man baby cakes."

She laughs. "Whatever…baby cakes."

I roll my eyes and put the box down. "I'm sure the lights are tangled, so get to work, woman, while I go grab the ladder, nails, and hammer.

"Should have done this part inside," she says as I walk around back.

*

Hours pass by, and I've hung enough lights to be able to see our house from space. We had all this last year, so luckily we didn't have to buy any new ones.

"Come on. Let's go get our tree," I call up to Sara as I warm my hands by the fire. They're stiff and burn like crazy. My gloves aren't worth a shit. She comes running down the stairs with a dark green sweater on that has a tree on the front and lights that actually light up. My wife is a Christmas tree.

"Let's go," she says, walking over to the coat rack.

"Hold up." I walk over to her and turn her to face me. "What the hell is this?" I ask, looking over her lights.

"It's a sweater, duh," she says, putting her arms through her coat.

"I know that, smarty. I mean, where did you get it and why?"

"It was on sale, so I didn't pay much, and why? Because Christmas! Come on, Cash. Get it together." She hands me my coat with a smile.

"You sure are chipper."

"It's Christmas!" she yells back as she walks to the truck, lights blinking as she goes.

*

We fire Old Blue up and head down the old country road that leads us to town. She sits beside me and wraps her arm around mine, making me listen to Christmas song after Christmas song. I pull up to the center of town and park the truck.

"So, are we getting a big tree or a small one?" I ask, already knowing the answer.

"Big." She smiles, and I take her hand as we exit the cab of the truck. We see the chief and Anne, and they walk over to us.

"Well, glad to see you two out and about on this pretty day," Anne says. She's in a red scarf, and a red knit hat sits on her salt and pepper head.

"It is a nice day," I agree.

"But cold," Sara says.

"You got a tree picked out yet?" the chief asks.

"Nope, just got here. Going to look around a bit."

"Okay, son. You two have fun. I'll see you at the office tomorrow." He nods his head, and I touch the tip of my ball cap as they make their way to his truck. I see a big tree on the back of it, and Sara grabs my attention.

"Let's go look," she says, tugging me. We walk through the trees, looking and handholding. Sara is so cute with the way she tries to decide on picking out one, so I pull her behind a big tree and sneak a kiss that takes her breath away. Her lips taste like cherry chapstick, and her blue eyes are glassy from the cold wind.

"What was that for?" she asks me.

"For being you." I smile and kiss the tip of her nose. "I got my Christmas tree. Let's go home," I say, looking down at her sweater.

She smiles and turns to look at the tree behind us. "Let's get this one."

"Okay." After we pay for the tree and have it loaded onto the bed of the truck, I spot Mark and Leigh walking toward us.

"You got yourselves a big one," Mark says.

"Sure do," Sara agrees.

"Nice sweater." Leigh smiles.

Sara smiles back. "It's Christmas, guys. When else can you wear a sweater like this?"

I kiss her hair, and Mark laughs.

"You know Bear still needs a good home," Leigh says.

"Who's Bear?"

Sara sighs. "A cute Lab that was found behind Banner's Bar." I nod when she answers.

"I'm getting in the truck. This wind is insane," Sara says. "Talk to y'all later." She waves.

Leigh looks to me. "She'd do great with a dog, Cash. You should come by and see him. He'd be a perfect Christmas gift for her."

"Now don't go making them feel like they gotta get him, Leigh," Mark says as I laugh.

"I'm just saying. He's smart, cute, and Sara seemed to like him."

"I may come down and take a look. We better get this tree on home."

Mark nods. "Talk to you later, man."

*

"Go open the door for me, baby," I say as we jump out of the truck. I grab the big tree and haul it inside, leaving a trail of green pine needles. I place the tree upright as Sara leaves the room. I hear Old Blue Eyes singing "Have Yourself a Merry Little Christmas," and my very own Christmas tree comes walking back into the room.

"Here," she says, handing me a beer. "I think we picked out a perfect one." She smiles as she goes to twist the cap off her beer. She fails and hands it over to me. I switch with her and give her my already opened one.

"I think we did, too." I put my arm around her and clink my beer against hers. "Here's to many more Christmases with you."

She smiles, and I look out the window and see the snow falling again. I take a swig of my beer and set it down on the coffee table.

"Is this where you want it?" I ask her.

"Yep."

I nod and walk over to throw a few logs into the fireplace before grabbing the box of lights and setting it beside my beer on the table. "Well, let's put some lights on it."

*

We put every ornament that we have on the thing. It's crowded, but Sara loves it, so that's all that matters. We sit on the couch with our feet propped up on the coffee table. A few empty beer bottles surround us, and Sara is cute tipsy. The old Christmas CD she has plays over and over, and the soft glow of the tree and the red flames of the fire are the only things that light the room. It's warm in here, and snow continues to fall slowly outside. I take my wife's beer from her hand and place it onto the table. She laughs because she's drunk, and I take advantage. "Let me kiss you."

"I'd never stop you." Her lips touch mine, and I taste beer, salt, and limes on her tongue. Crazy love likes limes in her beer and salt on her rim. It tastes good, and I want more. I push her back onto the couch and run my hand up her sweater, lifting it a little as my hand travels north. Our kisses grow more needy, and I climb on top of her and settle between her thighs. She wraps her legs around me, and I lift her sweater up and over her head, tossing it onto the floor beside us. I reach down and unzip my jeans, and she unbuttons hers and slides her zipper down. I lean back and grab the waist of her pants, yanking them off of her legs before I pull mine down. She grabs my neck and kisses me again. She's breathing hard, and I'm slipping her panties to the side, feeling her wetness. I grab myself and push inside. She moans into my mouth and bites my lip as I sink all the way in.

"God," she breathes as I move.

"Hold on to my hands, baby cakes."

She giggles and links her hands with mine. I put them above her head and move faster. The fire crackles and pops, and I hear the song from *A Charlie Brown Christmas* start playing as I love my wife in front of the tree I snuck a kiss behind earlier.

"I love you," I tell her. My voice is raspy, and I'm close to letting go.

"I love you forever, baby," she says as she falls, and I follow.

*

"Baby." I hear softly. My eyes open, and I see my wife. "Merry Christmas." She smiles like a kid, and my heart melts. I look over at the clock.

"It's awful early, girl."

"Or late, whichever way you wanna look at it."

I smile and roll over on my back, stretching as she climbs on top of me.

"Whoa," she says. "Someone happy to see me, or is that just morning—"

"I'm always happy to see you," I cut her off, and she leans down and kisses my nose.

"Up you get, husband." She jumps off of me and walks to the bedroom door. "I've got a few gifts under that kissing tree that have your name on them," she says before she disappears out of the bedroom.

I sigh and look out the window. It's frosted, and I see a heart has been drawn on it. "Crazy woman," I say, getting up and sliding my pajama bottoms up over my briefs. I walk to the bathroom and brush my teeth, smelling coffee and bacon as I do.

*

"What do you think?" she asks me as I look at my new wallet.

"I love it," I say, standing up.

"Where are you going?"

"I'm going to get my old one, so I can switch it out."

I hear her laugh as I run up the steps. Walking into our room, I grab my wallet from yesterday's jeans and walk back down the steps. Tossing my new wallet onto the table, I unload my old one.

"It's seen better days, hasn't it?" I ask her.

"For sure."

"Do you like your necklace?" I ask her. It's not much. It's small and dainty, and I got it at the pawnshop, but it's new to Sara.

"I'll probably never take it off," she says, holding on to the small heart pendant. I lean over and steal a kiss.

"I've got somewhere I gotta go," I say after switching my cards and old photo booth pictures of us from one wallet to another.

"Where?" she asks, like *really?* "Everything is closed."

"Just sit tight, okay? I'll be back." I kiss her nose and run back up the stairs to change clothes.

*

Ten minutes later and some serious questioning from my wife, I'm in Old Blue and headed over to Leigh and Mark's place. I pull into their driveway and put the truck in park. I see Leigh open the door, and in her hand she holds a leash, and connected to that leash is a brown-haired dog named Bear. He's the color of a grizzly and has kind, dark eyes. I step out of the truck.

"Merry Christmas," Leigh says.

"To you, too. Hey, Bear," I say. His tail wags, and Leigh gives me his leash as I lean down and pet him.

"Good morning." I hear and look up to see Mark on the porch with a cup of coffee.

"Morning. Santa bring you everything you wanted?" I ask.

He laughs. “I can’t complain.”

I nod. “Well, I better get back. Sara asked me twenty questions about where I was going.”

“Tell her Merry Christmas for us,” Leigh says.

“Will do.” I open the door and let Bear go first. He jumps right in, and I give Leigh and Mark a wave as I drive off.

“All right, Bear, I’m taking you to meet your new mom. Now, let me go ahead and tell you a thing or two about her. She’s got a big heart, loves hard, and has the prettiest smile you’ll ever see. Her curls sometimes bounce when she moves, and when she laughs it’s real. She’s going to love you hard, and you might help bring more of those pretty smiles she has. For that, I’m going to owe you. I’ll make sure to give you a treat every time. Deal?” He barks and nearly scares the shit out of me. I laugh at myself as I turn onto our road and head to our house.

I park the truck and see Sara come out the front door, barefoot, with her long gray sweater wrapped around her tightly. She squints her eyes and bites her lip. I open the truck door and step out. “Woman, your feet are going to freeze!”

“What do you have in that truck?” she asks on a grin.

"Come on out, boy," I say. Bear jumps down, and I hear Sara suck in air.

"Oh my God! Cash!" she says, running over to us. She leans down and rubs his face while he licks her.

"Come on, Sara. Your feet," I say. She hurries back inside, and we follow.

"Cash, you got Bear!'

"I got Bear."

"Aw, Bear. I'm so glad to have you." She smiles big, and he seems crazy happy.

*

Happy New Year hats sit on tables surrounding Banner's small-town bar while silver and black decorations hang from the ceiling. Champagne glasses are lined up at the end of the bar, and a local band plays on the stage. Sara's in a long black flowy skirt with a sparkly silver top that shows her stomach if she moves the wrong way. She says it's supposed to do that.

"You got one for me over there?" Mark yells to Banner, causing my attention to turn away from my wife's showing skin. He walks in with an arm draped over Leigh's shoulders. Banner smiles and grabs a beer from the cooler.

"You know I do, man." He places it on the bar, and Mark grabs it up.

"I'm starving," Leigh says. "I'm grabbing a few chips from the table over here. Mark didn't cook for me because he got off work late."

Sara laughs. "I'm coming with. Be back, baby," she says as she hops off the barstool and I see her sparkly top rise up again. Looking past her, I notice Ben walk in along with his date. Some girl he met around Christmas. He nods my way as she walks off to the restroom.

"You two a thing now?" I ask.

He shrugs. "I like her." He turns to Banner. "Hey, can I get two of those, Banner?"

"Sure thing," Banner says, reaching for two more bottles.

"How much longer we got?" Ben asks. I look at my watch.

"About fifty minutes. You guys are late for the party."

"You know girls, man. They take forever," he says, chucking his beer down. "You can go ahead and start me a tab, Banner."

"Will do," the bar owner says, placing Ben another bottle down. His girl walks out of the restroom and over to us.

"Boys, this is Shelby."

"Shelby, this is Mark, You've met Cash and the chief and his wife Anne."

"Hey," she says quietly with a small smile.

I nod, and Mark speaks, "What are you doing hanging out with this kid?" He grins.

"You aren't that much older than me," Ben says.

"Boy, I'm a good ten years older than you."

"No way. I didn't think you were that old."

"Hey, don't be calling me old now," Mark says, taking a sip of his beer. I grin, and Ben smiles down at Shelby. Maci walks out of the restroom, casting her eyes at me. I give a small wave, but then realize she isn't looking at me. I turn around and see she is looking at Banner. I look back at her as she heads over to the girls. Wonder what's up with that? I take a sip of my beer and look over at the chief. He's been nursing his for almost a whole hour, and that's not like him.

"You feeling okay, boss?" I ask.

"Yeah, just a little indigestion, is all," he answers, rubbing his chest.

"He's got bad acid reflux," Anne says. "He ran out of his prescription this morning, and the doctor is closed. His arthritis is also acting up."

"Now don't be telling them all my problems, Anne."

"I will because he asked," she says, taking a sip of her drink.

I chuckle. "You getting too old for the party scene, chief?"

"Son, I've been too old for it. I wish that damn clock would hurry up so I can get my ass to bed."

"Don't rush time, Drew. It already goes by too quickly," Anne says.

*

"You line it up with the ball, baby. Just like this," I say. Holding my wife from behind, I guide her pool stick, aiming it right where she needs to hit. "If you hit that spot right there, it'll go in that pocket," I say, pointing to the left corner.

"Okay," she says, smiling back at me. She pulls the stick back slightly and nails the cue ball, hitting the solid right where I told her. The ball spins and goes into the left corner pocket. She squeals and wraps her arms around my neck. "I did it, Cash."

"Yep," I say as she pulls back. "I'm grabbing a beer. Want one?"

"Please. I'm going to go sit with the girls for a bit."

I nod as I walk off to the bar.

*

Sara

Grabbing the party hat off the table, I place it onto my head and slide the thin band under my chin as I scoot in beside Maci. "So, what's up with those googly eyes at Banner lately?" I finally call my friend out as I wiggle my brows.

She laughs.

"Yeah, I noticed that, too," Leigh says, grabbing an olive from her fancy martini she had Banner make for her.

"I don't know what you two are talking about." But Maci blushes.

"You're blushing!" Leigh calls her out.

"I'm a redhead. We blush a lot."

"Nope, not true. My cousin is a redhead, and you can't get her to blush a bit."

"That's got to be a lie," Maci says.

"I've never seen her do it. Anyway, you're trying to change the subject. What's up with you and the bearded bar owner?" Leigh takes a sip of her drink and casts her eyes to me.

"Come on, Maci. Tell us something here."

Maci sighs. "Fine. I think he's cute, okay?"

Leigh gulps. "You think he's cute? Duh, he *is* cute, girl. Tell us something else! Why does he keep looking at you like he wants to pull on your ponytail and slap your ass?"

I burst out laughing. "Good God, Leigh."

"Too much?" Leigh asks, grinning from ear to ear.

"Both of you stop it." Maci is fire engine red.

I stop laughing. "Come on, Maci. We're just playing. We're happy for you. So, you're not talking to Lucas anymore?" I ask, serious.

"I was never talking to him. He wrote me, remember?"

"Yeah, but you told me you were confused back before Thanksgiving."

"Well, that was then and this is now. I'm no longer confused. In fact, I sent him the divorce papers again, and I told him it was over last week."

"Really?" I ask.

"Yes."

"Oh, Maci, I'm so sorry you had to go through all that bullshit," Leigh says, grabbing Maci's hand from across the table. "I know you did love him."

"Yes, I did love him with my whole heart, but it's done now. I'm moving on." She turns to face me. "Like you said, he treated me like crap, and you don't treat people you love like that. That is not love. I thought really hard about it." She looks over at the bar. "I thought so hard about it, actually on Thanksgiving, I came here and got cry-in-my-beer piss drunk."

Leigh laughs. "You did not."

"I did. Banner had to get me home." She chuckles a little. "It was embarrassing, but it happened, and the next day—minus the hangover—I felt really good about life again."

I give her a half-smile. "So that's why you didn't come to Thanksgiving."

She winces. "I'm sorry. I was just having a rough day."

"No, I'm sorry you were dealing with all that alone."

"She wasn't alone, Sara. Didn't you hear? The girl said she was here, with Banner!" Leigh winks, and I roll my eyes.

"You know what I mean. Does Banner not have any family?" I ask.

"He only has his dad, but I don't know too much else about him besides that."

"You plan on finding out, though, right?" Leigh asks.

"I hope so," Maci says, biting her bottom lip.

"We just want you to be happy, Maci, and if the bearded bar owner does it for you, then go kiss him when the hand strikes twelve," I say, smiling.

"I second that," Leigh says, lifting her glass into the air. She lifts it too high, and half of it spills out onto her hand and the table.

"Dammit, now I'm going to have to beg your boyfriend to fix me another," she says, sliding out of the booth.

"He isn't my boyfriend," Maci counters.

"Small technicality," Leigh says with a dismissive wave of her hand.

"He isn't!' Maci yells to her.

*

I grab my husband and take him out on the dance floor. He twirls me around and wraps me in his arms as we sway to the music from the band.

"Are you having fun?" he asks me.

"Yes." I glance over to see Maci talking to Banner, and I smile because I'm so glad my friend has chosen to move on with her life. Leigh and Mark dance beside us, and Anne got the chief up to dance, too. The music stops, and I turn to look.

"All right, everyone, the countdown begins!"

"Ten, nine, eight, seven, six…" we all say together. "Five, four, three, two, one! HAPPY NEW YEAR!"

Cash grabs my face and kisses me. I'm smiling, so he kisses my teeth before I can close my lips and kiss him back. I laugh when he pulls his lips away.

"I love you, baby. Here's to a great new year," he whispers into my ear.

Chapter Twenty-One
Cash

Icicles hanging from the town's trees start to melt as the snow also disappears. The sun shines bright in the vast blue sky and dries up the wet ground. The cold wind dies down and becomes warmer as winter finally fades to an end. Birds chirp happily from their nests as springtime flowers bloom. The days grow longer and the weather hotter. The boys and I play baseball again, and Sara has put back on her green floppy hat and got her nails dirty from digging in her garden. She and I visit the amusement park more, stuffing ourselves with cotton candy and greasy pizza. My amusement park buddy and Maci hosted another book fair at the library, and Leigh got some more pets adopted. Bear loves naps on the porch and his new home. We go for walks in the field, and he sleeps at the end of our bed.

The wife and I are sitting out on the porch swing sipping on lemonade she made earlier. It's cold and goes down well. The windows are up throughout the house, releasing baby blue paint fumes. She tosses the ball out into the yard, and Bear jumps up to go fetch it.

"Go get it, boy," Sara says. Bear grabs it in his mouth and runs back to us, dropping it back down in front of Sara. She picks it up and makes a face. "Eww, Bear, your drool is all over it!" He turns his head to the side, like he is trying to figure out what she's complaining about. Drool hater tosses it again, and Bear happily takes off. I take a sip of my lemonade and kick off the porch, letting the swing rock. Our dog drops the ball again, and Sara groans. "My arm is tired, boy. Cash, you throw it. It'll go farther." I drain the rest of my drink and stand, scooping the ball up before placing my jar onto the porch rail.

"Fetch, Bear," I say as I lean back and toss the ball across the yard. Bear barks and takes off. "That'll keep him busy for a minute," I say, looking down at Sara.

She smiles. "He's a good dog."

"He is a good dog," I agree.

*

I step onto the porch and stretch my legs. Sweat covers my brow from my morning run, and I wipe it before I head inside. I pass by Bear sleeping on the floor, and I hear him jump up and follow me up the stairs as I go to take a shower.

After my shower, I step over Bear and wrap a towel around my waist. After brushing my teeth and walking out to get my uniform on, I see Sara making the bed and humming to herself.

"What are you humming, baby?"

"'Lying Eyes' by the Eagles," she says, throwing the comforter up and smiling at me.

"Good song."

She nods in agreement, and I get dressed.

I place my ball cap on my head and slide my new wallet into my back pocket.

"You ready?" I ask my wife.

"Yeah," she answers, sliding her flats on and standing.

"Got a busy day at the library?" I ask as we head down the stairs. Bear follows us.

"Yeah, we have a lot of books to put up from the book fair we had. A library from the city donated a ton of almost brand new books."

"That's good," I tell her as I grab the keys to Old Blue.

"Yep." She leans down and kisses Bear's head, and I pat his back before we head out the door.

*

After I drop Sara off, I walk into the office and grab a cup of the finest coffee in town as Anne comes walking in from the back.

"Good morning," she says, but her usual chipper tone is not there.

"Morning, everything okay?"

"Ahh, Drew isn't feeling well today. I think he's getting a bug. You might have to take over for a bit. I'm sending him home," she says, taking off her reading glasses and pinching the bridge of her nose.

"Anything I can do to help? Want me to give him a lift?"

"Nah, I don't need you getting sick, too. I'll drive him. I told him to stay in bed. Old man never listens to me."

"I hear you yapping," the chief says as he walks over to us. He coughs and wipes his brow.

"You okay, chief?"

"Been better, son. I'm going to let Anne take me home. You keep an eye on things for me."

"Will do." I nod, taking a sip of my coffee. I look over when Ben walks in.

"Morning," he says with a rough voice. His hair is extra wild today, and he looks like he tied one too many on last night. He walks over to the coffeepot.

"What's with you?" I ask.

"I stayed up too late last night with some of my buddies from high school. I can't hang anymore."

I laugh.

"You shouldn't be staying up late knowing you have work in the morning," Anne says.

"Yes, ma'am," Ben agrees. "Chief, you okay?" he asks as he pours sugar into his cup.

"I'm heading home. Cash is in charge. Go check on the Kingsleys in a bit. Their neighbors called. Said they heard some yelling."

"We'll head on over there. Feel better," I say as they walk out. The chief waves his hand as Anne pushes him out the door.

"You're going to get in the hot shower right when we get home," she says before the door shuts.

"You ready to ride?" I ask Ben.

"I reckon."

*

As we make our way over to the Kingsley's house, I see smoke rising in the sky.

"You see that?" I ask Ben who has fallen asleep. "Ben, wake up," I say, hitting his chest.

"What?" he asks, jumping.

"Look." I point as we turn onto their road. "There's smoke, and it looks like it's coming from their house."

"What the hell have they done now?" He sits up and grabs his coffee. "My goddamn head feels like a hammer smashed it."

"What did you drink last night?"

"A little bit of everything."

"Don't you know mixing is the worst damn thing you can do?"

"I do now."

The Kingsley's house comes into view, and I see flames shooting up from the front yard. "What in the hell?" I ask, pulling into the driveway.

"She's set his damn chair on fire!" Ben says, jumping out of the truck. Elizabeth stands by, hands on her hips, as Joe, wet hair and no shirt, runs from the back with the water hose. I can't tell what he is saying, but from the looks of it, I'm going to need to handcuff him again.

Elizabeth looks over at us. "Well, boys, you've come just in time for the show. Joe here thinks he can sleep all day in this chair and not do any work around this place."

"You crazy ass damn woman!" Joe yells as he squirts the blazing chair with water.

"Well, you won't be sleeping in that chair anymore!"

Joe turns the water hose toward her, instantly drenching her to the bone. She screams as he laughs. I look over at Ben who is laughing, too. "Ben," I say under my breath. He stops. "Stop," I say to Joe. "Put the water hose back on the chair and get this damn fire out. Mrs. Kingsley…"

"Cash, I have told you…"

"*Elizabeth*," I say, correcting myself. "Get in the house." I point toward the house. She huffs and starts walking, dripping along the way.

"You two have to stop this mess. This is insane."

"I'm divorcing her ass. I've had enough."

"Not before I divorce you first!" she yells from the porch.

"Get inside before I arrest you for arson!" I yell back at her. "Joe, what the hell happened? How did she get this chair out here without you knowing?"

"I was in the bed asleep. She woke me with her loud ass yelling and slamming cabinets, so I finally got my ass up and took a shower. When I came out, the goddamn door was wide open, and I smelled smoke. She had already shoved the thing out here and lit the son of a bitch up. Elizabeth's stronger than she looks. She's been fussing at me for two days now. Saying I don't do anything around this place. Who does she think keeps the grass cut?" he yells as he puts his thumb over the tip of the hose, making the water come out harder.

"You two are going to drive me to drinking." I shake my head.

"Help yourself. There's liquor in the house. Hell, I shouldn't be the only one who gets to enjoy it. Gotta drink to be around her."

"I heard that!" she shouts from the door.

"Good!" he fires back.

"Get in the damn house!" I yell again. The door slams shut, and I lift my cap and rub my hair. The chair is only smoking now, and Ben looks like he could fall over.

"She's stubborn, isn't she?" Joe nods.

"You both are, and it beats the hell out of me why you stay married. Do you ever get along?"

Joe looks in front of him, wrinkles covering his forehead, and he shrugs. “Maybe when we first started dating, but for the most part, no. I love her, though. Would take a bullet for her if it came down to it. It’s just the way we’ve always been.”

“Well, it’s unhealthy,” Ben chimes in.

“Who’s to say anyone’s relationship is healthy? We all got our shit to sort. It’s not giving up on each other when the shit sorting gets tough—that’s what matters.”

I can’t help but crack a smile at Joe’s words. “You’re right, Joe. We all got our shit to sort.” I exhale and look back at the chair. “You need to come with me?” I ask.

“Nah, we’ll be okay. This just gives me a reason to buy a new chair. I’ve been needing one for a while anyway.”

I chuckle. “All right. You two behave.”

“See ya later, deputy.”

*

It’s nightfall, and the springtime breeze blows in from the field as I step out of my truck. I take my ball cap off and turn it around backwards on my head as I walk around the back and let the tailgate down, jump up, and take a seat. I reach into my pocket and pull out a cigar that the chief gave me. Lighting a match, I suck until flames fire up at the end and smoke drifts upward. The sky is filled with stars, and it's times like this that I'm glad to live away from the big city lights. I hear the screen door open then Bear's paws beating against the porch. I look down as he rounds the truck. He sits and looks up at me.

"Hey, boy."

He lifts up and puts his two front paws onto the tailgate. I rub his head before he falls back down. I hit my cigar as he lies at my feet.

"It's a good night to sit outside. Isn't it, Bear?"

He sighs and rests his head on his crossed front paws. The wind blows, making the branches from the big tree in the field sway. The leaves ruffle against each other, and it's the only sound to be heard out here. It's peaceful. It's the country. It's home.

"Baby?" I hear and turn to see Sara standing on the porch in her pajamas.

"I'm out here."

The screen door falls shut, and Bear's ears move when Sara comes near.

"What are you doing out here?" she asks me.

"Just enjoying the quiet. Come sit with me," I say and pat the tailgate. She steps over Bear and lifts herself up.

"It's pretty tonight." She sighs, and I take a hit from my cigar as we sit in comfortable silence and listen to the wind blow.

Chapter Twenty-Two
Sara

I laugh hard as I take off running throughout the house with Bear and Cash on my heels. I round the stairway and dart out through the screen door.

"Sara, I'm going to get you back!" Cash yells to me as I hear the screen door open. Bear barks. My bare feet move quickly over freshly cut grass, and in one swift moment, I'm flying and no longer touching the ground. Cash has me, and Bear runs around us in a circle, jumping and barking.

I laugh even harder as Cash wraps his arms around my waist tight and lets my feet touch the ground again. "It was just a little ice water." I giggle as he bites my neck.

"A little ice water?" he says. "It was a lot of damn ice water, and it froze my balls off. I have no balls now. Are you happy?"

I turn around in his arms and smile up at his handsome face. His hair is still wet from his shower, and he smells like fresh clean sheets drying on a clothesline.

"I'm sorry," I say, trying with everything to be serious, but the sound of his scream comes to mind and another laugh bubbles up.

"I don't believe you," he says, wide-eyed.

"But I really am."

"Sara!"

"Your scream," I can hardly say because I'm laughing so hard. "You sounded like a wounded animal." My eyes water, and my ribs ache.

"That's it," he says, lifting me up and throwing me over his shoulder.

"Cash!" I say, surprised, as I look at Bear upside down. Bear looks at me curiously before he barks again and follows behind us. I slap my husband's ass as he hauls me up the porch steps. I hear the door open and watch as we pass by the couch before he takes me up the stairs.

"Where are we going?" I ask.

"Our bedroom. I need you to find my balls."

I burst out laughing again, and he pops me on my behind.

"You're so romantic, baby," I tell him.

"Only for you," he says as he walks us into our room and shuts the door, leaving Bear out.

*

Cash

"How's the chief feeling?" I ask Anne as I take a seat across from her desk. She's got her reading glasses on top of her head.

"Still not great. The doc says he needs to stay in bed." She rubs her eyes.

"Anything I can do? Take him some soup or something?" I ask.

"No, son. Thank you, though. I'm keeping him drowned in soup." She sighs. "Once he is better, I'm sure he won't ever eat soup again." She laughs and puts her glasses back on. "Well, I've got some paperwork to get done here."

"And I've got some rounds to do. See you back here later."

She nods and looks over at the computer screen. I step outside, hearing the little bell above the door ring before I jump into my truck. I see Banner outside having a smoke, and I park the truck and hop out.

"How's it going, man?"

"It's going," he replies, taking a drag from his cigarette. "How's the chief doing? Heard he was sick."

"Yeah, doc has him on bed rest. Anne isn't giving a whole lot of details, though."

He nods and hits his smoke again. I turn to look at the small bar that seems like it's been here forever.

"How'd you come to own this thing?" I ask. He blows smoke from his mouth and flicks his ashes.

"Had some money put back, and I decided to buy this place." He shrugs. "Dad owned a bar my whole life. Guess I just felt like following in his footsteps." He kind of laughs, but it's without humor.

"What about you? Grow up wanting to be a cop?" he asks me.

I laugh without humor, too. "Just following in Daddy's footsteps."

*

Sara

I walk into the record store and look around. The smell alone tells me this place has been here longer than I've been alive. An older piano sits in the middle of the store, and music plays softly in the background. I search through boxes of old records and find a few I have to have. I take a seat on the floor and cross my legs, placing the records I want beside me.

"Let me know if I can help you with anything." I hear and peek around.

"I will. Thanks," I say to the older man who smiles and then disappears to the back of the store. I hum to the music, and my stack grows beside me as I slide across the floor and search through more boxes. I get up and walk around, looking through the shelves. I make my way over to the piano and lightly run my fingertips over the keys. My mom made me take lessons when I was a kid, so I can play a little. I sit down and let my fingers remember the old lessons. The door chimes, and I turn around to see my husband.

"Hey, baby," I say, smiling back at him.

"Hey, I saw Old Blue out there, so I figured you were in here," he greets me as I stand up from the piano. "Don't stand up. Play me something."

"Okay." I sit back down and inhale before I slowly exhale. I press the keys, and just like riding a bike, I remember the notes to "Can't Help Falling in Love". I sway as I play, and as I come to an end, I see Cash watching me. I drop my hands and stand up to face him. He reaches around me and presses down on a few keys.

“Falling in love with you was the best thing that ever happened to me,” he whispers.

“How can you say that?” I ask. His eyes dart to mine.

“Because it’s true. You’re my crazy heart.” He searches my eyes and looks down at my lips. Grasping the back of my neck, he pulls me to him and presses his lips to mine. He kisses me hard and backs me up against the piano, causing me to hit the keys. He grabs my leg and lifts it up around his waist as I rest my hands back on the old wood.

Pulling away, he looks down at me. “Come home with me,” he says, and I do. I leave my records on the floor and go home with my husband, because falling in love with him was the best thing that ever happened to me, too, and I love that I’m his crazy heart.

*

I’m lifted up as we enter our home and Cash carries me up the stairs. Clothes are taken off, and lips are kissed. Skin melts under skin, and sweet words of *I’ll love you forever* are spoken. Cash presses inside me, and I moan. The wind blows the curtains in the bedroom as he loves me. He grabs the headboard, and his teeth graze the skin on my neck. My hands fist the sheets, and sweet flames run up my spine as tingles of pleasure shoot down my thighs as I come.

*

I walk out of the grocery store with two loaded bags. The bottom falls out of one, and half of my crap rolls out onto the sidewalk.

"Dammit," I curse as I lean down and put the other bag on the ground. I chase an apple that's rolling, but it gets scooped up before I can grab it. I look up at the person who snatched it and see it's Cash's dad.

"Hey," I say slowly.

"Sara." He nods and hands me the apple.

"What are you doing here?" I ask.

"Can't come visit my son and daughter-in-law?" he questions as he leans down and helps me pick up the rest of my spilled groceries.

"Well, yeah, you can, Jack. But you haven't so…"

"I'm here now. You headed home with all of this?"

"Yes."

"I'd like to come along if that's all right."

"That's fine," I say as I walk toward the truck.

*

Cash

I park the cop truck and take a deep breath. I look over at his truck and grip the steering wheel. I wish I would have known he was coming. I would have drunk a few or thrown a couple shots back. It's been a while since I've spoken to my dad, and the last time was about as pleasant as a dog pissing in my shoe. My eyes look forward at the falling sun. Rays of light shine through the trees and make lines on the green cut grass. Dust particles fly around me, and I sigh as I remember back to the last time I spoke to my dad.

"So, you're moving, huh?"

"Yeah, Dad, we found a house, and we're buying it."

"You think that's a good idea? Taking her away like that?"

"I think it's best for us both to get away from here," I say, looking out at the neighborhood I grew up in. Everyone's house is decorated with Christmas lights, and it hasn't changed a bit since I was a kid.

"What are you gonna do when she goes through one of her fits and you're not there?"

"We'll figure it out," I answer him. He makes a noise that pisses me off. "It's obvious you don't approve of anything I do, so why can't you just keep your mouth shut? You like fighting?" I ask with a lift of my brow. Crossing my arms, I look ahead and clench my jaw. I see him look over at me in my peripheral. Ice hits the side of the glass as he takes a sip of the amber liquid he holds in his hand.

"You just need to use your head more, boy. You went and got married, without thinking it through, to a person you have to watch twenty-four seven. Now, you're leaving a good job and buying a house in another—"

I cut him off, "I've been with Sara since high school, Dad. What the fuck do you mean, I married her without thinking?"

"Don't cuss at me, son."

"You think I should have respect for you? You cheat on the woman you claim to love."

"That was a long time ago, boy, and none of your business." He gives me an icy glare.

"Oh, so it's none of my business, yet I'm the one who was here listening to her cry because you stayed out late 'working.'" I watch him down the rest of his drink before he turns to me.

"You do what you want, son. I'm done talking to you about it. Just don't come crawling back when it all goes to shit."

I watch him walk away with no expression on my face.

I shut the truck off and step out, getting ready for this shit storm that's about to take place. Walking up the steps, I see Bear. He pushes open the screen door and greets me.

"Hey, boy." I lean down and pet him before I walk inside. The house smells like food, which is odd. My woman can't cook well. I hear talking, and I make my way to the kitchen. My dad sits at the island with his back to me, and a drink on ice sits at the table. I see a bottle of his favorite drink on the countertop, and Sara stands at the stove.

"What's cooking?" I ask, surprising them both.

"Hey, baby," Sara says. Dad turns my way, and my eyes look to him and then back at Sara, whose eyes have grown wide. She makes a face.

I walk into the room. "What are you doing here?" I ask Dad while going over to the stove and giving my wife a kiss on the cheek.

"Wanted to come by and see how you two were holding up."

"Nice of you. We're doing just fine," I tell him, but then ask Sara, "What are you making, baby?"

"A chicken recipe Maci told me about. It seemed easy, so I thought I'd give it a try."

I give her a small smile and then turn back to my dad. Seeing the bottle on the counter again, I grab a glass and put some ice in it.

"Mind?" I ask him as I lift the bottle. He nods for me to go ahead. I fill my glass halfway and then go to walk out. "Wanna talk out on the porch?" I ask, but I don't wait for his reply. I keep walking until I'm at the door. Bear jumps up and follows me. I set my glass down on the porch railing and pick the ball up, tossing it far so Bear will have something to do. I hear the door open behind me. "Well, you've come. You see everything hasn't gone to shit, so…"

"So, what, you going to turn me away before I even get a chance to eat?"

"Sara's feelings won't be hurt. Like you care anyway, though," I say, taking a sip of my drink.

"Your mama misses you."

"You drove all this way to tell me that?"

"She wanted me to check in."

"Why didn't she come then?"

"I didn't tell her I was coming."

I nod. "You haven't changed. Still keeping things from her. You still messing around?"

"Son, I didn't come all this way to fight with you."

"I don't know why you came at all."

Bear runs back up on the porch with the ball in his mouth. He drops it, and I scoop it up, tossing it back into the darkness.

"How's she doing? I saw the scar on her wrist."

I look over at him. "She has her good days along with the bad."

"I told you, you would have to worry about this. One day she won't survive it, and then what's to become of you?"

"Don't you worry about that, and don't go killing my wife off just so you can get some kind of sick pleasure on being right."

"You think that would make me happy? To see you hurt and her gone?"

"Yes. You never wanted there to be a her and me anyway."

"I wanted better for you—yes, I did. Just like every parent wants for their child. She has problems, son. Ones you can't control."

"Like I said, we're doing fine."

Bear walks back up on the porch, and I go to the door.

"Have a safe trip home. I'll tell Sara you had to be on your way. Come on, Bear."

*

Later that night, a heavy rain falls, and lightning lights up the sky. I toss and turn in our bed until I feel tiny drops of water on my face. "Cash," Sara says. "I think the roof is leaking." More drops land on my face, and I sit up.

"Shit. Get up." I throw the covers off and step into a puddle of water. "Son of a bitch, there's water everywhere."

"I'll go grab some pots," Sara says. I move the bed under a spot that isn't dripping, and I sit down as Sara finds places to put the pots. "There are at least five spots."

"Yeah," I say, sighing.

"We're going to need a new roof."

"Yeah." I run a hand down my face.

“How can we afford a new roof?” she asks, getting back into bed.

“I’m going to have to get a loan. Don’t stress over it. I’ll figure it out.”

“You’re stressed. I can tell. If you stress, I stress,” Sara says as she wraps her arms around me. She kisses my neck, and I pull her on top of me. My hands move up her thighs, sliding her nightgown up her hips. I harden beneath her, moving one hand up to her breast and feeling its fullness. My other hand goes to her center, noticing she has no panties on. Thunder booms loud, rattling our windows, and I hear Bear move around at the bottom of our bed. Sara leans toward me and kisses my lips as I pull myself out and lift her up. She moans as she settles and slowly sinks down. Water drips into the pots surrounding our room, and the wind beats against the old boards of the house. I lift up as Sara goes down, and I grip onto her hips. Her head falls back, and when the lightning flashes, I can see her pretty face and the pleasure I’m giving her. I grab her hands, and she uses mine to help lift herself up. My body grows hot, and sweat forms on my brow. She lets go of my hands and removes her nightgown, showing me her gorgeous body. She’s been eating more, and she’s grown thicker. I love it, and I can’t keep my hands off her. I reach up and grab her breasts, and she sighs as her nipples harden beneath my fingertips. I lean up, running my fingers up her back, taking her nipple into my mouth. She cries out as she comes. I grip her shoulders, pounding upward, feeling my abs ache and tingles running up my spine as I groan out my release.

"Fucking hell, crazy heart."

"Cash, that was amazing." Sara lies down beside me, and I pull her close, as the storm keeps raging outside. Sometime later, her breathing evens out, but I'm wide-awake thinking how in the hell am I going to get this roof fixed. If I can't get a loan, I'm going to have to ask my dad. Son of a bitch.

Chapter Twenty-Three
Cash

With sweaty palms and shaky nerves, I sit across from the guy who will decide my future. He lifts his hand to his face and slides his glasses up the shaft of his nose with his middle finger after he looks up from the papers on his desk. They tell him how much I make a year and everything else he could possibly need to give me an answer. You know, my blood type, that kind of thing. I rub my hands over my jeans and take a look around me. Nodding to a few folks I know in the town, I look back at the man with the glasses as he clears his throat and removes the small frames from his face.

"I'm sorry, son. Your credit just isn't great, and with that house loan you've got here," he says, tapping his fancy pen onto the computer screen in front of him, "there just isn't anything we can do for you."

I lift my hat and run a hand through my hair. "Yeah, that's what they all tell me." I stand up, grab my papers, and put my hat back on.

"Check back in with us. Work on some things and then come back in here."

"I need this now or my roof is going to fall in." I turn away from him and walk out of the bank to get back into my truck. I toss the papers onto the seat, then crank the engine. Apparently, the idea of getting a bunch of credit cards when I was younger and not exactly paying them all has come back to bite me in the ass. We could ask Sara's parents, but that is just as good of an idea as asking mine. I make my way home, thinking I need to go ahead and give my balls away. I'll ask my dad for the money.

*

"There isn't anything else we can do?" Sara asks. We're seated at our supper table full of cube steak, gravy, and mashed potatoes. I take a sip of my beer and sigh.

"No, this is it. It's either I ask my dad or the next storm is going to cave our roof in."

"I know this is going to be hard for you, baby," she says, taking her feet off my lap and standing up. Bear's ears stand as she grabs her dish from the table. She kisses my head as she reaches over to grab my plate.

"That's an understatement. This is going to be hell. And he may not even give it to us." I take my hat off the table and put it on my head. "I'm pretty sure actually that he won't, but I have to ask him."

"I'll ask mine," she says, turning the water on.

"No, I can't deal with your mom's nagging. I'm sorry."

"Don't be sorry. I get it," she says, turning the water off and reaching for the dishtowel. She grabs the pots from the stove and scrapes the scraps into Bear's food bowl. He hops up and goes to check it out. I stand up and push my chair under the table, looking down at my dog as he gobbles his dinner. Sara walks over to me and wraps her arms around my waist. I lean down and kiss her neck as I snake my hands up the back of her T-shirt.

"It's all going to work out," I tell her.

"Sometimes I'm not so sure," she replies.

"Hey." I put my finger under her chin. "Don't think that way. We have each other. We'll be fine." She gives me a small smile, and I kiss her nose before I look over and see Bear is finished eating. "I'm going to take Bear for a walk."

She lets me go and walks back over to the sink.

"I'll be in the bath when you get back. I'm feeling achy today."

"Coming down with something?" I ask.

"No, just one of those days," she says more to herself.

I sigh. "Okay, we'll be back. Come on, boy." I push the screen door open and step out onto the porch. Sliding my hands into my pockets, I walk down the steps with Bear beside me. The evening sky shows the moon even though it's not completely dark out yet. "They say only a lazy man can see the moon when it's daylight, boy." He looks up at me. "You think I'm lazy?" I ask, patting his head. He sneezes, and I laugh. "Come on. Let's walk this food off."

*

It's the crack of dawn when I pull up to the house I grew up in. Even still, I know Mama is in there cooking breakfast and the coffee is ready. I take a deep breath and open the truck door. My boots sound heavy as I climb the steps I used to run down as a kid. I sigh as my knuckles tap on the door. A few minutes later, it opens and Mama is looking back at me. It's been too long since I've seen her. Her brown eyes have aged, and she shows more strands of gray throughout her once dark brown hair, but it's Mama.

"Cash?" she questions.

"Hey, Mama."

She opens the door. "Is everything okay?"

"Yeah, just in the neighborhood. Thought I'd stop by."

"Son, I might be a lot of things, but I'm not stupid. I know you were not just in the neighborhood at six in the morning. Come in," she says, moving so I can step by. I smell coffee, and I hear bacon sizzling in the frying pan. "Come on in the kitchen and have some breakfast. How's Sara doing?"

"Sara's fine, Mama."

"Have a seat. What have you been doing with yourself? You don't call. You don't come visit. You know I've been worried sick. I even asked your father to go check on y'all. He's a stubborn ass, though. Never does what I ask him."

I see he hasn't told her he came to visit.

"Been busy. Just trying to get in a routine."

"A routine? For six years?" she says sternly. "Here, have some coffee." She hands me a cup, eyeballing me as she does. I set it down on the table, looking at the steam floating up from the cup. She stands by the stove, and I can feel her looking me over.

"Mama, I'm sorry. I just couldn't get over the fact you and Dad didn't come to our wedding."

"I came," she says, causing me to look up.

"You came?" I ask, surprised.

“Yes, I couldn’t miss my son’s wedding even if I didn’t approve. So I came and stood outside the door.”

“Why don’t you approve? You know how much Sara means to me.”

She sighs and takes a seat down beside me. “I know you love her. A parent can’t help but want the best for their child, though. We all lived in the same town, Cash. The stories we heard about Sara growing up—she was troubled and wild. Unstable. Her own parents even had problems controlling her.” She gets up and goes to flip the bacon. “I see how much you love her, and I see now that we were wrong for being the way we were. I’m sorry. We were being judgmental, and we’ve wasted so many years.” Her voice breaks, and I see her shoulders shake as she puts the fork down. I get up and walk over to her.

“It’s in the past, Mom. Please don’t cry.”

“I’m just so sorry. So much time has passed. Six years I haven’t seen my son.”

I turn her around and wrap her in my arms. She hugs me back tight, and I feel like I haven’t been away from her for six years. I feel like it’s only been a few minutes, and I’m a boy again as I look around her kitchen. The kitchen she used to bake cookies for me in, the kitchen I’d have my after-school snack in, and the table I used to do my homework on. The room I told them I was going to marry Sara in, the countertop she placed me up on so many times after I had a wreck on my bike as she doctored me up. So many childhood memories in this house.

"I'm here now, Mom." I hear footsteps and look toward the living room when my dad walks in. He's dressed in jeans and a flannel shirt. His eyes land on us, and he gets a crease between his brows.

"Come to say you're sorry?" he asks, walking on in. Mama pulls away from me and wipes her eyes.

"Please don't start," she says. "Do you want some coffee?"

"I'll get it," he replies. I watch him fill his cup and put two spoons of sugar in it before he takes it to the table and sets it down. Mama smiles up at me and turns back to the stove. He walks by us and outside to get the paper I know is there. I inhale a small breath and walk over to the table while Mama finishes breakfast. Waiting for him to walk back inside, I take a sip out of my cup and look down at the table. I've got to get this out. He can either say yes or no.

"You seem like something is on your mind," Dad says. He walked back inside, and I didn't even hear him. I swallow before I go to speak.

"Dad," I begin before I lean back and lift my hat off. "I know we don't see eye to eye on things, but I'm asking you to put our differences aside for a minute."

He opens his paper and eyeballs me, eyes narrowed and lips in a straight line. "Okay," he finally says. "What do you need?"

"Jackson, who says the boy needs something?"

"Ruthie, he didn't come all this way for his health."

I look between him and her as he lays his paper down and his eyes lock on me.

"I need to borrow some money." He leans back and turns his head sideways, ready to speak, but I stop him. "Now, before you say no, I'll pay you back in payments and have you fully paid off within two years." I look over at Mama who flips the stove off.

"My roof is about to cave in. We had a bad storm, and now we've got about five good leaks in our bedroom and a few in the other rooms in the house. I've gone to the banks, but they can't give me a loan because of the house loan I already have, and my credit isn't exactly great."

Dad makes a grunting sound, like he isn't surprised to hear this. It pisses me off, but I swallow any feelings I have because I need this too bad to let my pride get in the way. He picks up his coffee and looks down at his paper as he takes a sip. I sit with a pounding heart and a knot in my stomach. If he doesn't give me this, I'll have to go to Sara's parents. God knows I'd rather crawl through a snake pit than hear Debbie's mouth.

"How much?" he finally asks as he puts his cup down. I'm shocked as hell.

"What?" I ask.

"How much? You didn't tell us a price. How will we consider it if we don't know what it is we are considering?"

I nod and tell him the price I got from the roofer.

"We don't have it," he blurts out with no thought at all.

"Now, Jackson—"

"We don't have it, Ruthie," he interrupts her. She clamps her mouth shut.

"I'm sorry, son. I told you when shit hit the fan, not to come crawling to me. Seems you got yourself in a bind, just like I thought you would, and I can't get you out."

I know he's lying. I know he has the money. My dad has always been a tight ass, but that's why he has money. That's why the bank gave me a house loan, just because they knew I was Jackson Williams' kid.

"Sorry you wasted your trip," he then says before he flips his page and straightens out his paper. Mama sets breakfast down in front of me. I stare down at it as she squeezes my shoulder and walks away. I'm not even a tiny bit hungry, but I eat it out of respect for her. Dad eats, too, and we sit in silence until we're finished. He gets up from the table. "Have a safe ride home," he says before he walks into the living room. I grab my hat and place it back on my head. Picking my dishes up, I put them into the sink and go to kiss Mama bye.

"I'll call more. I'm sorry it's been so long," I tell her.

She grabs me and hugs me tight before kissing my cheek. Her hand touches mine, and I feel paper. My eyes narrow in confusion, and she shakes her head and looks toward the living room. I tilt my head and look down at my hand. It's a check for a little more than I need.

"Thank you," I say quietly. She nods and goes to walk me to the door. She steps out with me and takes a breath after she shuts the door behind us.

"Your father has a lot of secrets," she says as she slides her small hands into her apron pockets.

I look down at the scar on her forearm from cooking fried chicken when she was a little girl. She told me about it one day after school. She said her mama was never home, so she had to learn to cook for herself. She knocked the skillet off the stove, and hot grease landed on her arm. Her voice causes me to look back up. "But I have secrets, too. You don't live with a man like that and not stash away some money just in case. He's a good man deep down, and I love him. I know he loves you and me. He just has a shitty way of showing it." She kind of laughs.

"We used to get along. I don't know what happened." I look out into the yard and shake my head.

"You decided to go your own way. He had a hard time with that, Cash. You're our only child…" She shakes her head. "We tried to make a good life for you. I don't know where we failed."

"Why do you think you failed?" I ask.

"Because you took off and never looked back."

"That had nothing to do with you or Dad. I needed to make my own way. I didn't want to be his shadow, and you said it yourself. Sara had a reputation here. We both needed a new start, away from here."

"Well, you did it," she says, looking away from me. I see her sigh, and I look at her face when she turns back. She gives me a small smile, causing wrinkles to appear beside her eyes. "Are you happy?" she asks me.

"I am."

She nods. "You take that money. Get your roof fixed and whatever else you need, but you make sure you call me and come visit. Bring Sara, too."

"Yes, ma'am. I can't thank you enough."

"I'm glad I was able to help. Take care, baby boy."

I give her another hug and head to my truck. Getting in, I turn back to look at her before I take off. She waves, and I lift my hand as I head back home with good news.

*

The workers get here at five a.m. every morning, waking Sara, Bear, and me. We're getting a brand new red tin roof, and the heat in the truck is getting fixed, too.

"Come on, Bear. Let's go for our morning run," I say, tying my shoes and standing. I kiss Sara's forehead. "We'll be back." She smiles and pats Bear's head before we take off outside.

"Morning, deputy." I hear as I come down the steps and look up.

"Morning. You boys need anything, you just ask Sara." I pick up my steps and start my run down our old road. It's peaceful this time of morning, but hell, it's peaceful here period. I get into a good stride with Bear running alongside me. My thoughts run, too, and I think about my mama and the money she let me borrow. I can't believe she had that much stashed away, and I bet she has more after all these years. I'm glad. My dad's a hard ass. She needs to protect herself, and it looks like she has. All those times she cried over him when I was younger—I always felt sorry for my mom and wished better for her. Now I see she has choices, and she isn't as stuck as I thought she once was.

I turn down into town with sweat dripping down my back. The sun is rising, casting a soft golden glow over the town of Green Ridge. I see stores starting to open, and once Bear and I make it to the small diner called Chevy's, I tell him to sit outside, and he does. I open the door, the air conditioner instantly cooling me off. Sliding onto a barstool, I grab the menu and look it over.

"What'll you have, Cash?" the waitress, Piper, asks me.

"The usual, please."

She nods, and I turn back to look at my dog who is sitting at the window looking in at me. I've been coming in here a lot lately after my run, so I've become a regular and so has Bear. Turning around, I see Piper has placed a bowl of water in front of me.

"He looks thirsty."

"I'm sure he is. Thank you," I say, grabbing it and walking it out to him. I open the door and place the water in front of him.

"Here you go, boy. Piper says you look thirsty." I pat his head as he laps up the water, and then I make my way back inside. A few minutes later, my food is placed in front of me, and I gulp it down before I throw some cash onto the counter.

"Thanks," I say before I head out.

Piper waves bye as she grabs my plates.

"Come on, boy. Let's get home so I can get ready for work." We walk back, and I see Anne opening up the office so we jog over to her. "Hey, Anne," I call out. She turns around.

"Cash, I tried to call you. I was hoping you were here. It's Drew. I've had to take him to the hospital."

"God, is he okay?" I ask.

“He was having problems breathing. The doctor said it’s pneumonia. Oh, Cash, I’m worried sick about him,” she says, resting her face in her hands. I reach over and hug her.

“He is going to be all right, Anne.”

*

But Chief Rogers was not okay, and only a few days later, pneumonia took him. We held his funeral the following weekend. The town of Green Ridge was devastated and so was poor Anne. It all happened too quickly. Even though he had been sick for a while, we thought he would get better. They say things work out the way they’re meant to even if it’s wrong. Well, I tell you this one was wrong. This place just isn’t the same without that old man.

The roofers will be finished with the roof today, and after my morning run with Bear and my breakfast at Chevy’s, I head back home to get changed for work.

Sara drives herself this morning, and I take my work truck. I park it and hop out, seeing that Anne has already opened the office door. The bell rings above me like it always does, and Anne looks up. She’s been crying.

"Anne, you don't have to be here. Ben and I can handle things."

"It doesn't matter where I go, Cash. He's everywhere. I have so many memories with that man."

I take a seat across from her and remove my hat. "Tell me about when you two first met," I ask. The town can wait for my rounds today. I'm going to sit here with this sweet woman and let her talk about the love of her life.

Her face lights up, and she grabs a tissue from her box on her desk. "Well, it was back in the sixties…" she begins.

Chapter Twenty-Four
Seven Year Anniversary

Cash

I walk out of the bathroom in a gray button-up shirt with dark jeans. Flipping the light off, I see my wife in a floor-length hunter green dress. I smile because she looks so good in green. She turns to face me as she puts an earring in her ear.

"You sure do clean up nice, Cash Williams."

"I do, don't I?" I look down at my outfit. She smiles and walks over to me. Kissing her lips, I wrap my arms around her and breathe in. "You smell pretty."

"Oh, I smell pretty, do I?" she asks, pulling away and giving me her smile.

"Yes, and you look pretty, too."

"Thank you," she says, looking into my eyes.

"Let's go eat, woman." I grab her hand and walk us down the stairs. I see Bear lying on the floor, and his tail slaps it with a hard thump when he notices us coming down. "Bear, hold down the fort. I'm taking your mama out for our anniversary." I pat his side, and we walk out the door.

*

Dinner is nice. We both order steak, but it's after dinner that I've been looking forward to.

We're driving down an older road, and Sara keeps asking where we are going.

"Just wait," I tell her.

She wiggles in her seat and looks out the window. It's dark, so she won't see what we are doing until we get there. A few minutes later, I'm pulling off the road and onto dirt. I look over at Sara.

"Cash, what could we possibly be doing way out here? I hope you aren't taking me camping. You know I hate bugs, baby." She looks out the back window into the bed of the truck, obviously looking for a tent. There are blankets and pillows back there, but no tent. "Why are there blankets back there?"

"Will you just wait and see, Mrs. Impatient?"

She huffs, but grins. Anne told me about this place. She said not a lot of people know it's back here. It's mainly for the people who just want to step back in time for a bit, and maybe relive their teenage years. The owners don't run it for the money; they have plenty from what I've been told. They do it for the memories. We round a curve and pull onto another small road before a huge field comes into view. I look over at Sara as she takes in the scene. I've never seen it either, but it's her expression I care about. Her eyes are wide with slight wonder, and her mouth is hanging open. Her fingers go to her lips, and she smiles.

"Cash." She looks over at me as I drive Old Blue forward and then back him up beside an old speaker.

"This is amazing. How did you find this place?"

"Anne. She said she and the chief used to come here all the time. They only play older movies."

"This is so cool. Like black and white movies?" she asks.

"No, I think newer than that, but they play those, too." I put the truck in park and open my door.

"Come on. Let's get in the back before the movie starts."

"What's playing?" she asks as she gets out, too.

"*Twister*." I smile.

"*Twister*?" She looks amused, but goes with it.

"Yep." I let the tailgate down, climb up, and reach my hand out for her to take it. She gathers her dress and takes my hand. I lift her up and tell her to get the blankets and pillows situated so I can go get drinks and popcorn. There are hardly any people here, and I think that's one of the best parts. You see, I've watched *Twister* a thousand times, but I haven't yet fooled around in the back of Old Blue. So if plans go the way I want them to, that's exactly what we'll be doing.

*

The movie is good, like it always is, and we've eaten all of our popcorn and put our drinks aside. I brought enough pillows to make us comfortable, and Sara is cozied up next to me as I draw small circles on her arm. We are the only vehicle on this side, and we're parked in the very back. I turn and surprise Sara as I move her dress up.

"What are you doing?" she asks me.

"It's our anniversary, baby," I say as I slip her panties to the side. She starts to protest, but my fingers enter her, and she can't help but moan. This makes my dick hard, and I scoot down more and put the covers over us. I make her feel good until she grips my arms and lets out a soft groan as she comes around my fingers. I climb on top of her while she is in a daze, and in one movement, my jeans are unbuttoned, and I'm slipping inside her.

Her head falls back, and I kiss her neck as I start to move, loving her in the back of Old Blue at a drive-in. I'd say it is bucket list worthy.

*

A few weeks have passed since our anniversary and I'm walking into the office with Ben, who is asking me what size ring Sara wears.

"Don't you think it's kinda quick to ask Shelby to marry you?"

"No, man. When you know, you know. You know?" he says, looking over at Anne.

"Boys, sit down. I have some news," Anne tells us. I look at her curiously before I take my seat. "The mayor has sent us a letter, and it seems as though you will be our new chief, Cash."

"What?" I ask, shocked.

"Yes, you will be our new chief. I've put in a good word for you and so did Drew before he passed. We spoke about it a while back, and he said that when he retired he was going to see if you wanted the job. The mayor and Drew were good buddies, went fishing together on the weekends more times than I can count, so the mayor said if you want it, the job is yours."

I look over at Ben who has a grin on his face.

"Dude, take it. I can't think of a better boss man than you."

I look back at Anne, who has a smile on her face, too, but hers is one of pride. This means a lot to her.

"That's some big shoes to fill," I say, looking down. "I don't want to disappoint anyone."

"You're the man to fill them. It's what Drew wanted," she says as her eyes glisten with unshed tears.

"Anne, I don't—"

"Think about it, Cash," she interrupts me. "Don't give an answer now. Go home, and talk about it with Sara."

I nod and look out the window.

"I'm going to go check on…something," I say just so I can get out of here. I get up and push the door open, hearing that bell ring above me just as it always does. I hop into my truck and head to I have no idea. I just drive.

When you're a kid, you have certain dreams. Some children want to be firemen, astronauts, teachers—hell, some even want to own a bar like their father. Me, I never had a clue, but I didn't want to be the sheriff or the chief of police. I worked with my dad to make money, so I could move away from that town one day and out from under Jack Williams' shadow. I accomplished my goal, and taking on the job as deputy here was just a way to hurry and earn some money for Sara and me. Now, I've got this big position thrown onto my lap and some pretty enormous shoes to fill. Drew was a legend around here. I'm no legend. I'm just a small-town boy who's in love with a wild girl. That's all I've ever been, and that's all I'll ever be.

*

"If you don't want to do it, then don't," Sara says to me as we walk out in the field behind our house. I've just cut the grass with a tractor I borrowed from Mark, and the wind keeps picking up chunks of wheat and tumbling them up into the air. Bear chases the windblown grass, but they only break apart when he sticks his nose in them.

"I just don't want to let anyone down."

"How could you possibly do that?"

I shrug. “If there’s a way, I’ll find it.”

“Cash Williams, you stop this self-doubt mess. If the chief thought you could do it, then you can.” She grabs my arm and turns me to face her. “You deserve this opportunity. You work hard, and everyone respects you around here. Make a name for yourself. I think you should do this. Grab life by the balls, baby cakes.”

I laugh. “Lord, woman, you sure know how to talk someone into something,” I say as I put my arm around her shoulders, and we start walking again. I reach down and grab a piece of wheat. Sticking it into my mouth, I look out at our land.

“I’ve been talking you into things almost our whole lives, baby. Why should I stop now?”

“I can’t find a reason,” I reply. “Guess I’m going to go for it. I’m going to grab this thing called life right by the balls.” I look down as she laughs. “Give me a kiss, baby cakes,” I say as I lean down and capture her sweet lips.

*

A Few Months Later

Cash

"Jesus, there's enough food here to feed a small army," I say to Ben.

"Well, it's not every day the mayor announces a new chief." He nudges my side and sticks a piece of ham into his mouth. I roll my eyes.

"Did you buy that ring?"

"Yes."

"When are you gonna ask her?"

"I don't have a clue."

I laugh. "Nervous?"

"Well, shit yeah, I'm nervous. Weren't you when you asked Sara?"

"No," I say in all honesty. "It wasn't planned." I look over at her laughing with Leigh and Maci. She's in a short brown dress with a black floppy hat over her pretty curls.

"Why did you two wait so long?" he asks me as he pops another piece of food into his mouth.

I shrug. "Just wasn't something we thought about or talked about. Thought maybe we'd be one of those couples who never got married, but just was always together. But married or not, I knew she was mine. Neither of us needed a ring or a piece of paper to prove that." I look back at Sara, and my mind takes me back to almost eight years ago.

I knock on Sara's parents' door before I slide my hands into my pockets. I hear heavy footsteps, the door flies open, and there's my girl.

"I heard you coming." I laugh as she jumps into my arms.

"Come on. Mama's driving me crazy," she says, grabbing my hand and nearly dragging me to my truck. I open the door, and she slides in first. Debbie runs out the front door.

"Sara! You put your seat belt on! Cash, don't keep her out too late."

"Yes, ma'am," I say as I shut the door and start the truck. Once we are out of her sight, Sara slides over and puts her feet on my lap.

"Good grief, that woman. She's been on my ass all day."

"Why?" I ask her as I drive toward the lake.

She laughs. "Because I snuck out last night and left muddy footprints on the carpet."

"You snuck out?" I look over at her with narrowed eyes.

"Yeah, I went to the water tower. Couldn't sleep," she says, wiggling her toes and yawning.

"Are you tired now?" I ask her as I grip her moving toes.

"Never too tired to hang out with you."

"Good."

I turn the radio up and roll my window down. The ride's only about twenty minutes, and as I turn onto the road, I look over at Sara who is sleeping. I don't wake her, because I know when she says she couldn't sleep last night, it means she probably didn't sleep at all. I drive on down and park the truck in the shade in front of the water. I gently move her feet off my lap, open my door, and step out. I grab my tackle box and fishing pole from the back and walk down to the water. After I put my bait on, I toss the line and wait for a bite. I watch the horseflies buzz above the water and the sun start to sink in the sky. I didn't plan to fish today, but with Sara I've learned you don't make plans because you never know what her mood will be. I'm okay with that, and really it's a good evening for fishing.

An hour later, the sun has completely set, and I've caught a few fish but threw them back. I hear the truck door open and look behind me.

"Baby, why didn't you wake me?" Sara says, stretching.

"You didn't sleep last night."

"But I wanted to spend time with you." She walks over to where I'm sitting on the grass and takes a seat on my lap. I wrap my arms around her and rest my back against the tree behind me. The oil lamp I bring with me for night fishing sits in the grass beside us and lights up her sleepy face. I look into her eyes, and it's as if the world stops spinning and nothing and no one but us matters. Her eyes are a pretty blue, her hair messy from sleep, and in this moment my heart feels completely full. She is all I'll ever need, all I'll ever want, and without any thought, I say something I had no intention of saying today.

"Marry me."

She smiles and leans back to search my face. After a moment, she says, "You don't want to marry me."

"I've loved you almost my whole life, Sara. If there is one thing I want to do, this is it." I tuck a stray curl behind her ear. "Marry me," I say in a rough whisper, almost pleading. She looks from my eyes to my lips, pulling her lips between her teeth before she looks back into my eyes.

"Okay," she whispers back.

"Okay?" I ask, unsure if I heard her.

"Yes, I'll marry you."

*

I step onto the stage after the mayor recites a long, nice speech in remembrance of Chief Drew Rogers and calls my name. The town cheers, and like my wife, I don't care for the attention, but I take a breath and look for her in the crowd. I find her and feel more at ease when she gives me a small smile and a little thumbs-up. I give her a wink and look back to the mayor as he says some more things about the town of Green Ridge and me. He then turns to me.

"Please, everyone welcome our new chief of police, Chief Cash Williams." I shake his hand, and he places the badge on my shirt. As the crowd cheers, I give a small awkward wave. He looks to me to say something, and I clear my throat as the crowd grows quiet.

"Hello, I'm Cash Williams. I'm honored…"

"Speak up, son," the mayor says, grinning at me. "They can't hear you."

I nod and clear my throat again, leaning into the microphone.

"Hello," I say louder. "I'm Cash Williams. I'm honored to be the new chief, and I'm proud that Chief Rogers picked me to follow in his footsteps. Thank you," I finish and hear one single person start to clap. I look and see it's my wife. Everyone soon follows, and I'm shocked Sara even singled herself out like that. I'm sure I'm grinning like an idiot, so I nod to the mayor and make my way off the stage, trying to get to her through the crowd. I spot her as she's making her way toward me. The mayor starts speaking again, and the town forgets about little ol' me. When Sara gets to me, she jumps into my arms and I kiss her hard, like no one is around. Pulling away, I smile at her. "You clapped first."

"Well, I couldn't leave my husband hanging after that awkward speech." She smiles. I think she's joking. I think. "I'm so proud of you, baby. You'll never know how proud I am," she says, holding my face in her hands. I kiss her again because I love this woman more than I love anything, and I don't care who sees us.

*

Chirping crickets, kids' laughter, and adult chatter fill the town of Green Ridge, along with hanging outdoor lights and candles lit on white table-clothed tables. It's been a beautiful night and the cleanup crew has started to pick things up.

Mark stands and taps a plastic fork against his bottle of beer as we sit outside Banner's Bar and watch the candles being blown out and smoke drifting upward into the night sky.

"That's not very loud, babe," Leigh says to her husband.

"It got your attention, though." He winks, and she shrugs, like *got me there*.

"Are you going to say something or not?" Ben says with a smirk.

"I'm getting to it," Mark fires back, but takes a sip of his beer. "Ahh, okay, where was I?"

"You were getting to it," Maci says.

"Right." He nods and clears his throat. "Hello, I'm Mark Phillips—"

"Shut up, man," I say, interrupting him and tossing an empty plastic cup his way. He ducks and laughs.

"No, man, seriously. I've known you for three years now, and I can honestly say there's no one better for the job of Green Ridge's new chief, and I'm glad to call you my friend."

I smirk. "Thanks, man."

"So, here's to Cash," Mark says, and everyone lifts their bottles and clinks them together.

"And more nights with good friends like you guys," I throw in before taking a sip of my drink.

"Come on inside, and I'll pour everyone a shot. We can toast it up right," Banner says as he stands up.

"Just one, though," Leigh says to Mark, "I've got a busy day at the shelter tomorrow, and you're already lit." She rolls her eyes as Mark stumbles inside. We all take a round of shots before everyone goes their separate ways.

*

I lift the covers for Sara to climb in, then wrap my arm around her waist and pull her up against me. "I love you, baby," I tell her before I kiss her neck.

"Love you more," she murmurs sleepily, and the noise of the rain starting to fall on our tin roof makes me smile with my eyes closed. I fall asleep to its comforting sound and my arms wrapped around my woman.

Chapter Twenty-Five
Sara

I'm hunched over with suds up to my elbows and a dog between my knees.

"Have you slept with Banner yet?" Leigh asks Maci as she squirts dog shampoo onto the Great Dane she's bathing. He shakes, causing most of it to come off. "Gosh dang it, Broozer. You've got to keep still or I'll never get you clean for your new family," she says, huffing and trying again to get the shampoo on him. "Well?" she asks Maci.

"Leigh, why do you want to know this?" Maci asks back as she wets her little furry I'm-not-sure-what-you-call-it dog down with the water hose.

"What do you mean why? I'm your best friend. I deserve…*we* deserve," she corrects, looking at me, "to know if you've slept with the guy or not." She's got bubbles in her hair from where Broozer decided he didn't want the shampoo on him again.

I lean up after I finish rinsing my dog off. "Guys, I've got to take a break. My back feels like it's going to snap in half."

"Mine, too," Leigh says, grabbing the water hose from me and rinsing what little suds off that she has on Broozer.

"You're bathing a Great Dane, Leigh. You don't even have to bend over," Maci says.

"Whatever. You still didn't answer my question." Leigh washes her arms off, and I reach over and get the bubbles out of her hair.

"Yes. I've slept with him. Happy?"

"Oh my gosh, you little whore!"

"*Leigh.*" I laugh as Maci looks over at her in shock.

"I'm kidding," Leigh says, holding up her hands. "Kinda." She winks at me and screams when Maci wets her with the water hose. She takes off running, and the dogs bark around her as Maci continues to follow her with the hose. I laugh until I can't anymore and Broozer takes her down and starts licking her face.

"Get off of me, you big ol' giant," Leigh says, kicking her legs out. Laughing still, I walk over and push the big dog off of her and grab her hand to help her up. She jumps up and looks over at Maci. "You got me. We are now way past even. Put the hose down," she says playfully. Maci nods, and I walk over and shut the water off. "Now that you have no weapons, tell me some details!" Leigh says, picking up the shampoo bottles and walking over to the pool deck. I take my shorts off and slide into the pool.

"I'm glad I wore my bathing suit," I say as I rest my elbows on the side.

"I'm getting in, too," Maci says as Leigh grabs her float and carefully sits down on it from the ladder.

"Details, please," Leigh repeats.

Maci sighs. "You two know I'd only ever slept with Lucas. I loved Lucas, and we had great sex—"

"No one wants to hear about the wife beater," Leigh interjects.

Maci looks over at her with wide eyes.

"Sorry," Leigh says. "I didn't mean it to come out that way. I just mean we want to hear about Banner."

Maci looks away, and Leigh makes a face at me, like *oops*. I roll my eyes and look back at Maci. "If you don't want to tell us, it's okay, Maci."

"Don't tell her that," Leigh complains.

"Anyway," Maci continues. "Sex with Lucas was always the same, but with Banner…" Her face turns red, and she grins.

"Oh my God. Are you in love with him?"

"Leigh, hush," I say. "Go on, Maci."

"It's just so intense, and there's so much…passion. Like I want to run as fast as I can and I also never want to leave his side. I don't know how to explain it."

"You really like him, huh?" I ask, smiling at her facial expression.

"I really, really do."

"I also did *you know what* in his truck, Leigh," Maci says, grinning with a super red face.

Leigh laughs. "Just like I said, little whore."

We all three laugh as Mark runs out.

"Cannonball!" he yells before he splashes into the water, soaking us all.

*

"What do you think, Bear?" I ask as I sit on the floor outside of the bathroom. I look at my watch and see that not much time has passed. I pet Bear as he lays his head on my lap. "Would you want to share us?" He makes a whimpering noise, and I lean down and kiss his head. "Don't be sad, boy. You'll always be our first." I stare up at the ceiling and sigh. Who knows, maybe this will happen, maybe it won't. I look back down at my watch and see that it's time. Moving Bear's head, I stand up, straighten my dress, and walk into the bathroom.

*

I walk out of the small shop and jump into Old Blue. It's a nice day, so I ride with the windows down and the radio up. I pull up to our house and hop out of the truck. Grabbing my bag, I jog up the steps and unlock the door. Bear greets me but passes by. Guess he has to use the bathroom. I sit down on the couch and take out my gift box and other purchases, hoping Cash will like this.

*

I've cooked the chicken recipe again that Maci gave me because Cash seemed to actually like it. Maybe he was just telling me that he liked it to not hurt my feelings, but he ate it all so… I stand up and put the dishes into the sink before I turn around to face Cash. "Have a good day?" I ask as he rubs Bear's head, and I rest my hands on the counter.

"Yeah, just visited the Kingsleys. Joe quit drinking."

"No way!" I say.

"Yep, says he's done with the bottle."

"Wow, well, good for him. What about Elizabeth?"

"She says one of them has to drink or they'll both go crazy."

I laugh and shake my head. "Those two need their own TV show."

"That's for sure."

"Did he buy a new chair?" I ask, walking over to grab more dishes from the table.

"Yeah, it's enormous, too. Elizabeth hates it, but she tells me she won't complain, because it's her fault he got a new one."

"I still can't believe she set his chair on fire. Come on, Bear. Let's go outside," I say and walk into the living room. I open the door, and he runs out.

"Trying to get rid of our dog?" Cash asks me as he walks up behind me.

"Of course not. I love our dog, but I have something to give you, so take a seat," I say, walking past him and opening the closet. I grab the box and turn around to see he is seated.

"What's this?"

"A gift. I bought it today." I hand it to him, then take a seat, too. I run my palms over my jeans as he looks at the box. He shakes it, but nothing rattles.

"What made you want to give me a gift?"

I shrug. "Just did."

He looks at me curiously before he lifts the top. I watch his facial expression as what I have bought comes into view. Confusion covers his handsome face as he picks the small clothing up and then looks over at me.

"Sara?" he questions as Bear scratches on the door. I swallow and take a breath as I get up and walk over to let him in. Bear wags his tail and goes past me to sniff what's in Cash's hands.

I lean my back against the door and bite my lip as Cash narrows his eyes and looks to my stomach. He stands up and puts the onesie down. Walking over to me, he rests one hand on the door above my head, and as he looks down, he places his other hand on my stomach.

"Are we going to have a baby?" he asks me in a low rough voice, sending chills all across my body.

"Yes."

He looks up at my answer and gives me a small smirk before he crashes his lips to mine. I'm thrown off, but I wrap my arms around his neck as he grabs my waist and pulls me closer. Breaking away, he searches my eyes. "Are you sure?"

"Bear and I have taken three tests that say so."

"How? You're on birth control."

"I stopped taking it."

"Without talking to me about it? I'm not mad. I'm just shocked and happy…really, really happy."

"I know I should have talked to you about it, but you know me. I just do things, and I figured if it was meant to be, it would happen."

"It's happened," Cash says. He smiles big and lifts me up into the air. "Bear, you're going to be a big brother." He kisses me again and steals my breath away.

*

Months Later

Cash

I open my eyes and blink. Stretching my arms, I roll over and look out the window as a soft breeze blows the curtains my wife hung last night to dry. The smell of clean linen fills our bedroom. I sigh, wondering where she is, so I get up. Placing my feet onto the hardwood floor, I run a hand through my hair and walk over to grab a T-shirt and jeans. I flip the light on in the bathroom and narrow my eyes. My heart starts pounding, and a bad feeling settles in my chest.

"Sara?" I call out, but hear nothing. I turn out of the bathroom, leaving behind an empty pill bottle with only half its contents spilled onto the floor. Sara's obstetrician doesn't want her taking any medication during her pregnancy. He says some women have healthy babies while on their bipolar meds, but some do not, so we don't want to take the risk. These pills shouldn't even be here. I jog down the stairs, calling her name again, but still no answer. My hands start to shake as I search through every room of the house. "Where is she?"

I step out onto the porch and see the truck is gone, too. Bad thoughts run through my mind as I look on the side of the house. My heart swells, and I almost cry. There she is. Standing beautiful with her pretty green hat on. Her very pregnant belly is underneath a long dress. Bear is lying beside her feet, and Old blue is parked by her garden. She's planting more flowers. I sigh in relief and step off the porch to make my way over to her. Bear's tail starts to wag, and he lifts his head.

"Hey, baby." She smiles.

"Hey, crazy heart." I smile back. I slide her hat off and kiss her lips, her nose, and her forehead.

"What was that for?" she asks.

"I missed you," I tell her. She's glowing, and her blue eyes are the color of the sky above us.

"You missed me?"

"Yes," I say, kissing her again and wrapping her in my arms. She giggles and makes my heart swell more. God knows I love this woman more than my own life.

"Did you have a good nap?" she asks me as she wraps her arms around my back. Her stomach is in the way, but I love her stomach.

"Yeah. What's up with the pills on the floor?" I ask, pulling away.

"Oh, Bear's tail knocked them off the shelf. I was looking for that foot lotion I bought, and he was right up my butt. I could only get so many of them up because of Little Miss here." She smiles, rubbing her belly. "I went down to get the broom, and I got sidetracked."

"What did you do with the ones you picked up?"

"I flushed them, crazy. I'm not going to take pills that have been on the bathroom floor."

"Oh, that explains it." I sigh.

"You okay?" she asks, looking at me like I've lost it.

"Yeah, I'm good. Did you go buy more flowers?" I change the subject.

"They had some on sale down at the hardware store, so I got Mark to put them on the back of the truck for me. I just got home not too long ago. Bear rode with me, of course. He won't let me out of his sight." He lifts his head at the sound of his name. Bear is always around Sara now that she's pregnant. I'm pretty sure he will be stuck up Little Miss' butt, too. "You wanna help me get these big pots off the truck and onto the porch? I thought it could use some color."

"I'll take care of it. You go make us some lemonade," I say, kissing her forehead and walking over to the truck.

"Gladly. My thighs are sweating," she says as she wobbles toward the porch.

*

Sara's water broke at five a.m. this morning, and at one p.m. Little Miss' first cries were heard throughout the fourth floor of the hospital. We named our baby girl Ellie. She weighs no more than a feather to me, and I am terrified to hold her. Afraid she may crumble in my arms, I sit in a rocking chair now, smiling down at her sleeping face while Sara sleeps, too. It's just us three right now. Everyone has been by, held her, and gone home. Ellie moves her little hand, and her mouth opens a tad. I look at her patchy reddish skin and run my finger along her small nose. Her hair is so blonde you can hardly tell she has any. She's just peach fuzz and little round cheeks, red lips, and tiny fingertips. My heart could explode with the amount of love I already have for her.

*

"Are you sure I can't stay and help out? Dealing with a newborn isn't easy, Cash, and Sara seems to be sleeping more so than anything."

"Debbie, we're fine. Go on home to Walter. We'll call you if we need anything."

She sighs and looks back up the stairs where her daughter sleeps. Her granddaughter is in my arms, and I'm pretty sure she wants her to leave, too.

"Okay, but what about her medication? The doctor said she needs to start back taking it. We have to watch her. She has a high risk of postpartum."

"I've got it," I tell her as I hold my little football and open the door for Debbie to exit. She looks at the door and then at me.

Defeated as always, she sighs. "All right." She leans down and kisses Little Miss before looking back up at me. "Cash, you have to watch Sara's moods. I'm worried about her getting postpartum. She could very easily fall into a depression, and we both know it."

"You've said that already. I'll watch her, okay? Have a safe trip home."

"All right. I'll talk to you later. Bye, Ellie."

I watch Debbie walk out the door, and I look down at my baby girl.

"Grandma is a tiny bit overprotective, Little Miss. But you'll learn that later," I say, walking into the kitchen. I grab a beer and Little Miss a bottle before I head back to the couch and we catch up on some sports.

*

"Cash, baby." I open my eyes and see Sara looking down at me, realizing I must have dozed off. I sit up and run a hand over my face. Sara has Ellie, and she's dressed in a different nightgown, meaning she must have taken a shower.

"Hey," I say, sounding groggy.

"You were sleeping well." She sits beside me.

"I was tired, I guess."

"I'm sorry I've been MIA."

"I'm not complaining." I grin playfully.

"You love spending time with our Little Miss?"

"Of course, she's my new sports buddy."

"You better not turn her into a tomboy."

"I'm not making any promises," I tell her. Sara smiles and then sighs as she looks toward the muted TV. "How are you feeling?"

"Better. I think I was just worn out. I know it's been a few weeks since we left the hospital, but it just took a lot out of me. Thank you for being so supportive."

"I'm just taking care of my family, Sara."

"I know, but you really go above and beyond. I'm a lucky girl."

"You are." I wink.

*

We sit outside on the porch swing while Ellie sits in her own little swing. Her blue eyes are wide as she stares at Bear who stares back at her. He won't get too close just yet, but he is always near, making sure Little Miss is safe. I put my arm around Sara and kick off the porch.

"Do you think she is going to look like you or me?" Sara asks me. "It's just too early to tell right now."

"Hopefully you. She has your eyes already and your blonde hair."

"Yeah, but her hair could darken."

"True."

"I wonder what kind of personality she is going to have. What she is going to like to do and what she will think is funny."

"Me, too," I say, looking over at Ellie. She does nothing but lie there, swinging and watching everything, but it's the most entertained I've been in a while. "I could watch her all day."

“I could, too,” Sara says, laying her head on my shoulder. I link my fingers with hers and bring her hand to my lips, kissing it lightly before resting it back on my leg.

“I love you.”

“I love you, too,” she says, giving me a smile.

Chapter Twenty-Six

Five Years Later

Cash

Fog rolls past the trees and sweeps across the street. Early birds wake and deer run wild through the woods, while the road winds and my feet hit the pavement. The sun lightens the sky, but hasn't shown yet. Sweat slides down the side of my face, and my thigh muscles ache as I make it into town. Bear stayed home, sleeping beside Ellie's bed so it's just me out here this morning. Sara stayed up all night and finally laid down as I was lacing up my shoes. Her eyes were closed when I left, so I'm hoping she'll be ready for Little Miss' birthday party this afternoon.

I stop running once I get closer to Chevy's, and I stretch before I walk in the door and feel the air conditioner.

"Morning, chief," Piper greets me, setting down a glass of water as I slide onto a stool.

"Morning."

"Where's Bear?" she asks.

"Can't get him to come with me anymore. He stays with Little Miss."

Piper smiles. “That girl is adorable.” She slides her hands into her apron pockets and leans her hip against the counter.

“She looks like her mama,” I say.

Piper nods in agreement. “You want the usual?”

“Yep.”

*

I’m showered and dressed for work when Sara walks out of the bathroom in a towel and wet hair. “Sleep okay?” I ask.

“Kinda.” She sits on the bed and grabs her lotion from the nightstand. Little Miss walks in with sleepy brown curls and no shirt. What can I say? She’s got a little bit of me in her.

“Good morning, baby girl,” Sara says, and the smile on Ellie’s face constricts my heart. She runs over to her mama and jumps into her arms. “Did you sleep well?” Sara asks Ellie as she kisses her all over her face. Little Miss giggles, and I don’t want to go to work today.

“Somebody turns five today,” I say, getting my girl’s attention. She looks over at me and grins.

“I do, Daddy.”

“Yep, you’re one whole hand now.” I hold up all five fingers and walk over to her. She reaches her arms out for me to grab, and I swing her up into the air, blowing kisses on her little belly just to hear her laugh more. I look down at her mom, seeing she is smiling at us. I then hear Bear as he walks in. Ellie wiggles her feet to get down, so I let her.

“Bear, you snore, but I love you,” Little Miss says as she gives him a hug. Sara gets up and walks to the closet to find some clothes.

She no longer works at the library, choosing to stay home with Ellie now. I make more money as chief, and I’ve paid my mom off so we are doing better than we once were. Life has been okay. Sara went through a little postpartum, but the doctors expected it. We were prepared, and we got her through it. She still has rough times where she can’t seem to get out of bed, and Ellie doesn’t understand why her mommy doesn’t feel well a lot or why she gets mad easily, but all in all Sara is great with her and I see how hard she tries to stay focused and keep her emotions on track. She still visits Dannie and takes her medication like she should. We haven’t had any scares over the last five years, and for that I thank God every day.

Sara grabs her clothes and walks into the bathroom, only cracking the door so she can get dressed.

"Let's go downstairs and I'll make you some breakfast," I say to Ellie as I lift her up from behind.

"Come on, Bear," Ellie demands. "You've got to eat your breakfast, too!"

*

"Look, Daddy. Bear likes cereal just like me and you." Ellie laughs as Bear licks out of her bowl. I shake my head and walk over to the table.

"He has his own food, Little Miss," I say, taking it away from him and putting it in the sink. Ellie makes a sad face.

"But he likes it, Daddy."

"He likes a lot of things," I tell her and look up when Sara walks in. She has a white tank top on under some black overalls, and she has tossed her curls up.

"What are you girls going to do today?" I ask.

"Today, we are going to the library for story time," Sara answers excitedly to Ellie. "Does that sound like a fun time to you, Little Miss?"

"We going to see Aunt Maci?" Ellie asks.

"Yes." Sara grabs the coffeepot and her mug. I hand her the cream and grab my ball cap from the counter.

"Well, I guess I'll see you two later. I've got to check on the Kingsleys. Anne has already called and told me their neighbors have been calling in. Ben is still at home with Shelby and the new baby for a few more days, so it's just me."

"Tell them hello for us," Sara says.

"Will do." I kiss her lips quickly and then kiss Little Miss before I head to the door.

*

I park my work truck in front of the office and step out, giving a few folks a wave before I step inside, hearing that same bell that's been above the door for longer than the eight years we've lived here.

"Good morning," Anne says, looking over at me. She stands over her green flowing flower with a watering pot in her hand and her reading glasses sitting on top of her gray hair.

"Morning," I say, walking over to the coffeepot and filling a cup. You can't come in here and not have a cup of Anne's coffee.

“Did you run this morning?” she asks me as she moves to another plant.

“Yep.”

She smiles and tilts the pot. “I ran across an old photo this morning of Drew in high school. He was so good-looking,” she tells me. “Sometimes I miss him so much I have a hard time breathing.” She stops watering and puts the pot down. “I forget that he’s gone even after five years, Cash. Last night I decided I wanted a sandwich, so I went into the kitchen to make it, and then I thought to ask him. I actually started to say his name.” Anne looks down and takes a shaky breath. When she looks back up at me, her eyes have glossed over. “And then I remembered and I cried like it happened yesterday. I didn’t eat the damn sandwich. I came up here and sat in his office.” She casts her eyes down the hall and shakes her head. “Your office now, which you haven’t changed a bit,” she says, looking back at me.

“It’ll always be his office. I can’t change anything in there,” I say, sliding my hand into my pocket and taking a sip of my coffee.

“You’ve only added a picture of you three.” She smiles. “How’s Little Miss doing today? It’s her birthday, right?”

“Yes, it is. She’s a happy little girl. Going to do story time with Sara at the library.”

"That's good. Kids need to read more books. They're too busy with their video games these days."

I nod and put my coffee down. "So, what about the Kingsleys? What are the neighbors saying?"

She shakes her head and rolls her eyes. "You'd think after all these years those two would calm down. I thought once Joe stopped drinking they finally would."

"Well, it has been a while since we've been over there."

"You're right. It may just be Elizabeth's pregnancy hormones. I still can't believe they are having a baby."

"Not just one," I say.

"No! *Twins*?" Anne asks with wide eyes.

"Yep. They found out last week. I saw them coming out of the doctor's office. Joe was white as paper, and Elizabeth had a wrinkle between her brows. I stopped and said hello. Elizabeth turned to me, and with a concerned expression, she said, 'Twins.' And then she started fussing at Joe about how he had to give her twins. Couldn't just be one baby, but two. How they couldn't afford diapers for two babies."

"What did you say?"

“I didn’t say anything. I drove off.” I laugh.

“Oh, Cash,” Anne says, slapping my arm as she laughs, too.

*

I pull up to the Kingsley’s place like I have a million times before and shut the truck off. I see a big box that’s been thrown out into the yard and on it is a picture of a crib. Walking past it, I step onto the porch and knock on the door. Elizabeth opens it moments later.

“Cash, what can I do for you?” she asks, smiling like the sun never goes down and it’s always a perfect seventy degree day.

I narrow my eyes and adjust my hat. “Just came to see how you guys were doing.”

“We’re just fine. Would you like to come in? I’ve got some chocolate chip cookies that just came out of the oven.”

My eyes grow wide, and I’m not sure if I’ve stepped into the twilight zone or if this is actually the Kingsley’s house. I want to touch her forehead and make sure she hasn’t come down with some deadly fever.

“You made cookies?” I ask.

"Yes," she says, looking at me. "Come in," she insists so I do. I step inside and smell the cookies. I hear an electric screwdriver and see Joe in the middle of the living room with a big ass crib. He notices me and stops his work.

"Cash, how the hell are ya?" he asks, putting the power tool down and standing up.

"I'm doing well. Just got a call from your neighbors earlier. I came to see if everything was okay."

Joe shakes my hand, and Elizabeth shoves a tray of cookies in my face. I look from it to her before I take one. I'm still confused as shit. It's like an episode of *Leave It to Beaver* without the Beav. I'm looking at Ward and June instead.

"Oh yeah, we got into a little argument over this here crib. You see, I bought the wrong color," Joe says, taking a cookie for himself. Elizabeth walks back into the kitchen, and Joe leans in. "She gets a little nuts sometimes. I think it's the hormones," he whispers, looking over my shoulder. "I told her I'd paint the thing after she got done screaming at me and tossing the box out into the yard. You see it when you walked up?"

I nod.

"She did that," he says, taking another bite. "That's a big ass box, Cash, but she threw it like it was nothing. It still had parts of the crib in it. I had to go outside and fetch them."

"You two want some milk?" Elizabeth asks. Joe, wide-eyed, looks a little terrified that she might have heard him. I'm still in the twilight zone.

"I'll take a glass," he says, then looks at me, nodding for me to get one, too.

"Umm…me, too, thanks," I say, still looking at him. He smiles big and goes back to the crib. I follow.

"Joe?"

"Yeah, chief?"

I lean in like he did to me. "Are you scared of Elizabeth?" I ask quietly.

He laughs like I'm crazy for saying that, so I laugh a little, too, but stop as his face grows serious. "Cash, she threw a box full of crib parts out into the yard. One minute she's baking cookies, the next she turns into the damn Hulk. Wouldn't you be a little scared? She has two humans growing inside her that are probably going to be just like her. I'm scared to death and the happiest man on the planet at the same time."

I nod my head at his smiling face and put the rest of my cookie into my mouth before I pat him on the shoulder. Elizabeth hands me the milk, and I down it.

"I'm going to get going now. Elizabeth, thanks for the cookies and milk. Joe, I'll see you later," I say as I hand her the cup.

"Anytime, Cash," she says, smiling and putting a hand over her stomach. I walk out and shake my head.

Everybody in this town is having babies or losing their damn minds. Hell, some of them are doing both, I think to myself.

*

I step out of the truck with more balloons than the movie *Up*. Tables are set up outside in the front yard, and my little five year old is standing on top of a chair with a red cape on her back. "Daddy, look. I'm Superman and I can fly!" she yells before she leaps and spreads her little arms out wide. She has blue lips from the Popsicle in her hand. I tie the balloons onto the side window of my truck before she runs over to me and jumps into my arms. "Did you bring all those balloons for me?" she asks.

"Yep." I kiss her cheek and look up when Leigh walks out of the house. "Come on, Supergirl. Your mama wants you to change your shirt."

"What's wrong with my shirt?" Ellie asks, looking down. It has blue stains all over it.

"Looks like you got a little dirty, Little Miss."

She giggles. "Daddy, that's not dirt. That's Popsicle."

"Oh, right," I say, kissing her again and moving her brown hair from her shoulder. She looks like her mama in almost every way, has her blue eyes, her pretty face, and her fun personality. But she has my brown hair, and she likes doing what Daddy does—fishing, playing with Bear, and watching sports. She's a little Sara and a little me all in one.

*

A few kids run around us screaming and blowing bubbles while Mark and I sit on the porch steps nursing the beers in our hands. Sara sits with Leigh and Maci out at one of the tables as Anne talks to my mom. I look over at my dad who is chasing Little Miss around the yard. She has two balloons tied to her wrist, and Sara put her hair up into some kind of messy something. It's falling all around her face, and she swipes it out of the way as she runs from her grandpa. He catches her, though, and lifts her into the air. I can't help but smile as she laughs.

We've come a long way. We still don't see eye to eye on everything, but these past years have been good…better I should say. I hear the door open, and Banner walks out with Ben's kid.

"How in the hell did I end up with a newborn? Where are this kid's parents?" he asks, walking past us.

"Ben and Shelby snuck out back, said they were giving you some practice." I laugh.

"I'm not having kids, so I don't need the practice. He keeps making a weird face, man. You think he's pooping?"

I lift my chin, looking at the kid's face. "Yeah, that's definitely a poop face."

"Fucking hell. I'm going to find those two. I don't give a shit what they're doing. I'm not changing a brown diaper. I'll throw up, man. I've got a weak stomach." He gags. "I smell it," he says. "I fucking smell it." He walks off with Mark and me laughing.

"Cash, where are the birthday candles? Don't y'all think it's time for us to do the birthday cake?" Debbie asks. I look back.

"Ask her mama," I say, taking a sip of my beer.

"How many of those have you had? Do you think you should be drinking at your daughter's birthday party?"

"Debbie, this is my damn house. If I want to drink a beer, I will."

She huffs and lets the door slam behind her.

"You do seem a little drunk off that one beer you haven't even finished," Mark says with a grin.

"Shut up," I say, downing the rest.

*

After the birthday cake is passed out and the presents are opened, my daughter smiles big with icing on her face as my mom snaps a picture of us three. Bear eats his own plate of cake, and Little Miss gets down from her chair and runs over to Walter. He lifts her up and bounces her on his knee.

"Pa, your mustache looks like a caterpillar. Will it turn into a butterfly?" she asks him. I don't hear his answer because my attention turns to Sara who appears to be fussing with her mom. I tell a few people bye as they leave and take their kids with them. My eyes look toward the porch, and I see Maci and Banner swinging. Those two have been together for a long time now. He still hasn't asked her to marry him, but I think she is okay with that. Lucas did a number on her. He got out a while back I heard, but I never told her. I'm not sure if she already knows or not. He hasn't shown his face around here, so that's all that matters. I feel a pat on my shoulder and look back to see my dad.

"Your mama and I are heading out. Thanks for inviting us."

"Of course." I nod and stand to give Mama a hug.

"Love you, baby boy. We'll talk later this week," she says, giving me a kiss on the cheek. I shake my dad's hand before they go over to tell Ellie bye. My eyes go back to Sara who is shaking her head. She throws her hands up like she is defeated before storming off into the house. Mama looks her way after she puts Ellie down. She looks back to me, and I give her a small smile. She doesn't return it. She looks worried, and I don't like it. I clear my throat and walk past Debbie who has taken a seat.

"What did you do to piss her off?" I ask low enough for only her to hear.

"She's not taking her medication, Cash."

"How do you know this?" I ask.

"I looked in her weekly medicine container. It's slap full. Don't you check these things?" she asks like she didn't do anything wrong.

"What the fuck are you doing snooping through her stuff?" I ask.

"Cash," Walter warns.

"No. You don't go into someone's house and look through their shit." I speak louder than I should have.

"I was just looking out for my child because obviously her husband doesn't."

"That's enough," I say. "You need to go, Debbie. The party is over, everybody."

Leigh now has Ellie, and she's crying. Leigh nods at me, letting me know she's got her, so I head inside to find my wife.

"Be gone when I come back." I look behind me to say to Debbie.

The screen door slams hard when I walk in and I hear Maci tell Banner to help her clean up.

"Sara," I call out. I hear nothing, so I walk through the house in search of her. Seeing she isn't downstairs, I run up the steps. Walking into our bedroom, I turn the corner to see Sara sitting on the floor. Pills are scattered around her, and the bathroom mirror is cracked. Blood covers her knuckles as she grips onto a fistful of her dirty blonde curls. Her shoulders shake from the sobs coming out of her mouth, and her head is down.

Like the mirror, my heart cracks at the sight of her. "Baby?"

She looks up at me with tear-stained cheeks. "I hate her," she says, crying more. I walk over and sit down on the floor with her. When I pull her to me, she switches her blonde curls for my shirt, and it soaks up her blood and tears. "I hate her, and I hate taking that fucking medicine."

I don't say anything; I just let her cry it out. Looking up, I see Maci standing at the doorway. I shake my head at her, like *not now*. She nods and reaches for the door to shut it. I know I can trust those people down there with my child, so I don't question where Ellie is. They're family and love Little Miss as much as her mama and I do.

My ass is numb, and Sara has finally calmed down enough for me to pick her up. Once I do, though, I notice she has fallen asleep. I cradle her to me and kiss her forehead before I walk over to the bed. Laying her down, I lift the throw from the bottom of the bed and put it over her. I look at the rise and fall of her chest before my eyes lock on her face. Her lips are slightly opened, red and puffy like her eyes were when I walked in.

Debbie's words pass through my mind. She is right, though. I should have looked myself. I don't understand why Sara stops taking her medication, knowing it helps her. But maybe they don't. I don't know. She has changed medications so many times. She's tired. She's tired of it all. Looking down at my T-shirt, I see blood and wet spots from Sara's tears, so I lift it up over my head and grab another one out of the closet before I walk out of the room, leaving her to rest and making my way down the stairs. The front door is open, and I look out the screen and see Leigh and Maci sitting on the front porch steps with Ellie.

I hear her talking, so I listen. "Mommy gets sad sometimes," she tells them. "I always give her a hug when I see her crying. It helps. I thought." She's still wearing her red cape on her back, and little curls fall from her pulled up hair. She puts her elbows on her knees and her cheeks on her little closed fists. I slide down the wall and rest my forearms on my knees. My heart falls in my chest as I listen to my little girl tell our friends the sad truth about her mama. I lean my head back against the wall, looking up at the ceiling, remembering the day Sara and I painted it white more than five years ago.

"My arms are so sore. I won't be able to lift a toothpick," Sara says. White drops of paint are all over her old overalls, and she's barefoot with baby blue toenails. I smile at her because she looks so damn beautiful right now I can't imagine anything prettier.

"What are you staring at?" she asks, giving me a grin.

"You."

"Why me?" She climbs down from the ladder and lays her paint roller down onto the paint tray. She wipes her forehead with the back of her hand before placing both hands on her hips.

"You're so goddamn beautiful."

"Cash." She smiles. I walk over to her, and she drops her arms. As I look into her eyes, she laughs.

"Why are you laughing?"

"Because you're being all sappy again," she tells me.

"Oh, I'm being sappy?" I ask her playfully.

"Yes," she says, shaking her head and placing her hands onto my chest. I surprise her and lift her up. She grins wider before she takes her bottom lip between her teeth. I kiss her, making her let it go. Dropping to my knees, I lay her down on the old sheets we have on the floor that catch the paint droppings. She smells so good and tastes even better. I run my hand up the side of her body, making my way up to the clasp on her overalls. I unhook them, and they fall behind her back onto the floor. She slides them down, and I lift her shirt up. Going down, I kiss all over her stomach, then help take her pants off. I hook my fingers into her

panties, and they go, too, before I make quick work of undoing my pants.

She's naked on our living room floor, and I'm still fully dressed. I pull myself out and line up at her entrance. She's soaked, and I moan as she surrounds me. Her legs snake around my waist, and I cover her lips again with mine as she slides my baseball hat off. I make her groan, and she drives me crazy when she runs her hands through my hair. She's my sweet thing, my life, my fucking crazy heart, and I make her see stars as a strong wind enters our house through every open window. It blows the sheets around us, and Sara's body lifts up toward me as she comes and tells me how much she loves me.

Chapter Twenty-Seven
Cash

I throw the line into the water and set my pole down so I can help Little Miss throw hers out.

"Is Mommy gonna be okay?" she asks me.

"Yeah, Grandma is home with her."

"She seems so sad, and I think I should be there with her."

"Well, Mommy wants fish tonight, and Daddy needed a fishing buddy."

"Okay," she says. After I put her line in, we take a seat on the ground and look out over the water. "There's another fisherman over there, Daddy," Ellie says, pointing.

"Yep, he's gonna catch him some dinner, too."

He walks closer to us, and my wild child yells at him, "Hey! What's your name?"

"Ellie," I scowl.

"I'm just saying hey, Daddy."

"You know you aren't supposed to talk to strangers."

The man turns toward us, and I see who it is. He doesn't look at me, only at Ellie. "Name's Lucas," he says. "What's yours?"

"Mine's Little Miss," she says proudly. "He's not a stranger now, Daddy." She grins at me.

"Pick up your pole, baby girl."

"But what about the fish?"

"Do as I say. Now," I tell her. She pouts, but does it anyway. "Go on and get in the truck." She doesn't question me this time. "Lucas, what business you got coming back here?" I ask, walking over to him.

"Well, deputy, I didn't realize that was you there. You got a little one now?" he asks, looking past me at Ellie.

"You need to be getting on your way."

"I don't think that's something you can decide. I think I'll stay. I've always liked this little town. Plus, I need to pay a visit to a long-lost wife of mine." He grins before he leans down and spits in the dirt.

"You get on out of here, Lucas, or I'll have no choice but to bring you in. This is your one and only warning."

He laughs. "What? You gonna tell the big bad chief on me?"

"I am the fucking chief," I say, surprising him by grabbing the front of his shirt. His eyes grow wide. "And if you don't get the hell out of my town, you'll wish you never came back." I toss him away from me and he stumbles backward. "Don't let me see your face again." I turn away from him and walk back to my pole. I grab it out of the water and toss it into the back of Old Blue before I get inside.

"Daddy, who was that?" Ellie asks.

"A mean man you won't be seeing again." I crank the truck and look over at him walking back to his car. I don't move until he drives off down the road that heads out of town. I say that to Ellie, but I know he'll be back. I put the truck in drive, and we make our way into town to pick up some fish from Sally's Market.

"What are we gonna do about Mama's fish?"

"We're going to buy some."

"Will they taste the same? I don't want her to be sad."

I chuckle sadly. "They'll taste the same, baby. Don't you worry about Mama."

*

"How's she feeling?" I ask Mama when I walk into the house.

"She's sitting out back, said she wanted to get some air," she tells me as she takes the groceries from my hands. "You didn't catch any fish?"

"Nah, ran into a little issue, no big deal, but we ended up going to buy some instead."

"Well, I'll cook it up. Come on, Little Miss, and help Grandma cook."

"Thanks, Mama," I say, walking over to the fridge. I grab a beer and head toward the back door. I step outside, hearing the nighttime bugs and seeing Sara sitting at the table we have out here. She's facing away from me, but I can see that she rests her chin on her bent-up knee. A gray sweater covers her arms, and her hair is wild as it falls around her back and shoulders. I sigh and walk over, taking a seat beside her on the bench. She doesn't even look over at me, and I see the tiredness in her pretty face. I lift my hand and move her hair away from her shoulders so I can see her face better.

"Baby," I say. I see her swallow before she looks at me. She gives me the smallest smile before she turns back toward the field. "I saw Lucas earlier."

"What?" she asks.

"Yeah, I told him to get the hell out of here." I take a sip of my beer. "I hope he listens."

"I hope so, too," she murmurs. I hear the back door open, and Little Miss rounds the table.

"Mommy," she says, grabbing Sara's leg. She hugs it hard, and Sara puts her hand on Ellie's back.

"Hey, baby. Did you have a good time with Daddy?"

"Yes, but we saw a mean man and Daddy told him to go away. So we didn't get no fish. But we went to Sally's, and Daddy paid for them instead. He said they'll still taste the same, Mommy, so don't be sad."

"Okay, sweet girl."

Ellie removes herself from Sara's leg and climbs up on the table. "Look at those lights out there," she says, pointing toward the field.

"Those are fireflies," Sara says.

"If you run inside and ask Grandma to give you a jar, we can go catch some like Mommy used to do when she was a little girl."

"Catch them?" Little Miss asks. "But how will they breathe?"

"We can put holes in the top so they can breathe."

"Okay," Ellie says, jumping down and taking off toward the house. Sara stands up and she and her bare feet walk out to the field. She stands there watching the fireflies while I sit and sip on my beer watching her. Little Miss runs out of the house, passing by me, heading straight to her mama. She tugs on her sweater and hands her the jar. I see Sara wipe her face, and I know she has been crying. Why is she so sad? I just don't understand it. Ellie doesn't notice, and Sara unscrews the top before handing it back to her.

She points out to the field for Ellie to run and try to catch them. I lean back on my elbows, watching my pretty girl with her long brown hair as she goes in circles. My eyes look over at my wife holding her face, and I see her shoulders shake. I take a big gulp of my beer and cast my eyes to the sky, taking in the enormousness of it and all the pretty stars. I see a shooting star, and it reminds me of the time Sara sat on my lap and asked me if I wished for babies. I didn't wish for babies then. I wished for the same thing I'm wishing for tonight—for my wife to be happy and for her to never leave me.

*

"Yeah, he was fishing at the pond Ellie and I always go to," I tell Ben as we sit at Chevy's eating breakfast.

"Son of a bitch. I can't believe he's back in town," Ben says as he takes the last bite of his eggs.

"Well, he is and we got to go tell Maci and Banner, just so they can be prepared. I know he'll be back." I lift my finger for Piper to bring me the bill so we can leave.

*

We pull up to Maci's house and climb out of the truck. The smell of smoke hits me immediately, and I look over the hood at Ben.

"You smell that?" I ask.

"Yeah, smells like something's on fire." I look around, trying to find out where it's coming from, and when I look back toward the house, I see it.

"Fucking hell, Ben. Call the fire department!" I yell back at him as I take off running toward the house. I try the knob, but it's locked, so I rare back and kick it in. Smoke rolls out in waves, and I lift my shirt to cover my nose.

"Maci!" I call out.

"Cash!" she yells, but I can't see anything. It's too smoky, and my eyes start to burn.

"Maci, where are you?"

"I'm in the back bedroom. I can't get out. The fire is blocking the door!"

I hear a gunshot, and I know it came from the backyard. Looking down the hallway, I see the door is wide open and flames crawl up the wall right in front of Maci's door. Another gunshot goes off, and I start to panic.

"Shit, Ben. Maci, you're going to have to break the window! I'm coming around. You'll have to jump out!" I hear the fire trucks coming down the road as I run out of the house. I look for Ben but don't see him anywhere. "Ben!" I yell. I run to the back of the house and hear a loud crash as something goes through the window along with heavy smoke.

"Cash!" Maci coughs.

"Come on. You've got to jump. I'll catch you."

"I can't. I'm scared."

"Maci, you either jump or you're going to die. You don't have a choice," I say, holding out my arms. "Come on. I've got you!" I need her to hurry.

I've got to go find Ben. She looks back into the house before looking down at me. "Maci, come on!" I yell.

She grips onto the side of the window just as I hear the fire department pull up. A few men run around the house as she steps onto the windowsill.

"Step back, chief. We've got her," one of them says to me. I nod, stepping back.

"Maci, they have you. I've got to find Ben." I run toward the woods, but look back to make sure she got out. The men catch her as leaps out of the window.

"Ben!" I look all around, seeing nothing but trees. My eyes search everywhere before landing on something. It's two somethings. I run over and see Ben and Lucas lying on the ground. Ben groans, holding his side.

"Ben," I say, leaning down. "Have you been shot?" I look at his side, noticing blood. I lift my radio and call for an ambulance. I know the firemen have medical equipment, too, so I whistle and yell their way. "Ben, keep pressure on it. They're coming." I stand up and look over at Lucas. He lies flat on his stomach. I walk over and put my finger against his neck. He has no pulse, so I lift his shoulder.

"He's dead, chief," Ben says painfully. "I saw him running out toward the woods. I chased him and tackled him from behind. The son of a bitch had a gun, and he shot me when we rolled over. I was able to pull mine out just before he went to pull the trigger again. I shot him in the stomach."

The firemen run over to us with their medical equipment as I drop Lucas' shoulder.

"See to Ben," I tell them.

*

After I talk to the fire department about how they think Lucas started the fire, I tell Ben I'll check in on him later as the medics shut the ambulance's doors and drive him away to the hospital. I turn back just as the mortuary service zips up the body bag that holds Lucas. They load him up, and I walk over to Maci who is sitting on the porch steps.

"You should have gone and gotten checked," I tell her.

"I'm fine, Cash," she says. I sit down beside her and take my hat off.

"How's Ben?"

"They say he is going to be okay, looks like it just grazed him good." I run a hand over my beard and look down. "What the hell happened?" I ask as I look over at her.

"I saw him a few weeks ago."

"What? Why didn't you tell me?"

She shrugs. "I don't know. I was shocked and scared. I thought maybe my mind was playing tricks on me. It was only the back of his head, but I knew it was Lucas. I just knew it. I've been going crazy ever since. I was going to talk to you at Ellie's birthday party, but all that happened. It's been more than five years since I've seen him. Why would he come back?"

"He was a fucking psychopath."

"I don't understand it. I don't know how he changed so much." She wipes a tear from her face, leaving a trail of smut from her hand. "He made me lose my baby, Cash. We were arguing one night after he came home from Banner's shit-faced. I packed my things to go stay with my mom just until he sobered up." She rubs her nose and looks down. "I was walking down the steps here, and all of a sudden I was shoved from behind. I fell down face-first. It knocked the breath out of me, and I woke up the next morning in our bed. There was blood, and the doctor confirmed what I already knew. My baby was gone."

"Why didn't you press charges against him?"

She sighs and picks at a loose piece of wood on the step. "You know people say they would have done this or that," she says, looking out at the yard. "But that's so easy to do until you're the one living the nightmare. I loved him." Her shoulders shrug like it's the only answer there is, like it's enough. Love can make you do things you never would, and it can make you put up with things you shouldn't. "He promised he would change, Cash. He told me he didn't mean to push me. That he tripped over his own foot and fell himself, and that's why I fell," she scoffs and shakes her head.

"So he lied about it."

"Yeah, he lied and lied again. Things only got worse after that. He didn't change. I think the guilt he felt from making me lose our baby overtook him." She breaks the small splinter away from the porch step and tosses it. "He started drinking a lot more. I could deal with him sober. He didn't push me around, but drunk Lucas was a whole other person."

"The fire department says the fire was started from gas and a tossed cigarette. Did he smoke before?"

"He must have started like I did a while back." She shrugs. "I quit so I didn't have any in the house." Maci runs a finger across her lips, and a wrinkle forms between her brows. "I knew I felt someone watching me. I was asleep, but even still I had a feeling. I thought it might have been Banner, but he left earlier to go meet an inspector at the bar.

I woke up because my nose was burning from the smoke."

"I'm just glad we came when we did."

"Me, too, Cash." We both look when a car pulls into the driveway. Banner jumps out and runs over as Maci stands.

"What the fuck happened?" he asks her. "Are you okay? Did he hurt you?" He grabs her arms and looks over her face.

"I'm fine, baby."

"Cash, thanks so much, man. I don't know what I would have done if…" he doesn't finish his sentence. I stand and shake his hand before I pat Maci on the back.

"I'm gonna go. I'll talk to you two later. Take her to the doctor if she starts having any trouble from the smoke, Banner."

"Thanks," Maci says as I put my hat back on and make my way to the truck. I get in and see Banner with his arms around Maci. I'm glad she has him.

Chapter Twenty-Eight
A Few Months Later
Sara

I watch as tiny dew droplets slide down the grass blade in front of me, like a teardrop falling down someone's face. My body aches, and I roll over and look up at the sky. I'm all over the place again. My mind runs in circles, tiring my body out, but not shutting down long enough for me to sleep. The days and nights all feel the same. I've felt like this before. My daughter is at school now. She started a few weeks ago, and I now have too much time on my hands. Cash is busy, but I keep him busier with my shifting moods and sudden outbursts. I think he would be better off without me. I would like to shut down and not feel like this anymore. An airplane flies over me, and I lift my finger and close one eye, covering the silver speck in the sky, thinking we are all just tiny specks.

*

It's two in the morning, and I know this because I stare at the clock beside our bed. I've watched it since it was ten. Cash sleeps beside me, and I roll over and look at his handsome face. I love him so much—him and Little Miss, but these thoughts I'm having are going to take me away.

*

I crawl into bed with Ellie and breathe her in. Her sweet smell gives me comfort. I kiss her dark hair and scoot down so I can see her face. She's beautiful. The most beautiful thing I've ever done, and I know she will be an amazing woman. She's smart and witty. Her presence alone lights up a dark room.

It's five a.m. now, so I get up because she will be waking in a few hours to get ready for school. I kiss her one more time and climb out of bed. Bear lifts his head, and I lean down and pet him. "You watch after her always," I say. "Always, always."

*

I sit on the porch swing watching as the sun makes its first appearance, brightly declaring a new day. I rest my chin on my knee and look over when I hear the front door open.

"Hey, baby," Cash says as he leans down and touches his toes.

"Hey."

"You okay? Did you sleep?" he asks me.

"Yeah, a little," I lie so he won't worry. I'm so tired of making him worry. He walks over and leans down. Taking my face, he kisses my lips. I close my eyes and savor his touch. Tears build up behind my eyes. He lets go, and it was too quick.

"Love you. I'll be back."

"Love you, too," I say as he jogs off the porch. The tears fall down my cheeks, just like the dew that slid down the grass blade, and I sniff and wipe my eyes before I go in to get Little Miss ready. I climb the steps with no energy, and once I make it to the top, I sigh and stop for a minute, looking down into our living room. The old broken house we turned into a beautiful home. A home full of memories and struggles, happy times and sad ones.

Love.

Love is what makes a house a home. But hope is what makes life worth living, and I've lost any that I may have had. I run a hand through my hair and walk into Ellie's room.

"Little Miss," I say quietly. "Come on, sweet girl. It's time to get up."

She rolls over and blinks her eyes open. "Can I stay home with you today?" she asks me. "We can sleep."

I smile. “You have to go learn something new. Come on. Up, up,” I tell her as I walk over to her closet. “Dress or pants today?”

“Pants every day, Mommy.”

“You don’t like your dresses?”

“Not really. I can’t crawl good in them. My knees get all scruffy.”

“Well, we don’t want that.” I smile a little before getting her outfit and helping her in it. “Raise your arms,” I tell her. She does, and I take her pajamas off and slide her shirt over her head. I kiss her nose once her shirt is on. She reaches up and rubs my cheek, surprising me.

“I look like you, Mommy?” she asks.

“I think so.”

“Good,” she says before she stands and we put her jeans on.

*

I’m kissed goodbye, and I watch as my family walks out the door, leaving Bear and me alone. They wave with happy smiles, and I walk out onto the porch and take a seat on the step. Bear sits beside me and rests his head on my lap. I pet him and mindlessly stare out at the yard, not thinking about anything in particular and everything at the same time. I lean my head against the porch rail and close my eyes. Over time, we will be nothing but dust. Forgotten as the wind tosses us about. We will forever fly, but forever be no more.

Chapter Twenty-Nine
Cash

The bell dings above me as I walk out of the office door and grab my keys out of my pocket. I turn around and lock up for the night, looking up at the sky as I do. It's dark for this time of day, and I feel like a storm is coming. Leigh called me earlier and said she was going to grab Little Miss from school. She has a few dogs she needs help with and she wants to spend some time with Ellie. So I climb into my truck and head to Billy's Barbeque to pick up dinner.

I'm walking out when I hear the ambulance coming through town and I wonder what could have happened now. I jog to my truck and jump inside, setting the food down in the passenger seat. My radio goes off, and I hear my address and the police code 10-56. My hands shake as I grab my keys and shove them into the ignition, yanking the gear shifter in drive and turning my emergency lights on. My tires spin, and I leave smoke behind me. I don't stop once.

The ambulance is already there when I pull up, but the medics are just now opening their doors. I jump out and run toward the house, seeing

Debbie's car parked and Walter standing at the door. I look at him as he steps in front of me.

"Cash."

"Move," I say as my voice breaks.

"Son, you…"

"I said fucking move." I shove him out of the way and rush past him, taking the stairs two at a time. I pass Bear who has his head resting on his paws. He's whimpering. Debbie sits on our bed, gripping the comforter under her hands and staring straight ahead. I swallow and turn to see the bathroom door cracked with claw marks at the bottom. I push it open more and see the blood first. My knees buckle from under me, and I hit the floor. Crawling over to her, I reach for her and press her pale face into my chest. I look down and see her arm, so I grab her blood-covered wrist and hold on to it, trying to keep the blood from pouring out. The sound that leaves my throat is unrecognizable, and the pain that slices through my heart makes me question if it's still whole. I rock her and kiss her soft curls.

"You promised, baby. You promised," I cry as the medics come inside and pull me away from her. I rock as though she is still in my arms. I cry, I rock, and I die inside.

*

Chaos and machines with loud beeping surround me. People rush past me, and questions are thrown at me from everywhere. "I don't know," is all I can say, because I don't. I never knew. It was a battle I was never a part of. It was all Sara.

"We're losing her." I hear and the beeping stops, turning into one long sound. "Time of death." I look over at the doctor as he announces it and I rush out of there, running as fast as I can until I burst through the doors. I lean over and throw up, hurling toward the ground and holding myself up by my hand on the wall.

"I told you!" I hear from behind me. I shut my eyes and stay put. "I told you she would do this! You didn't watch her! You were never there," Debbie cries, and my shoulders shake. She walks over to me, and I falter sideways when she shoves me. "You were never there!" she screams and starts hitting me. I let her because I need to feel something else besides this pain that's ripping me inside. She screams more and cries harder, hitting my back, shoulders, and slapping my neck and face until I finally grab her and put my arms around her tightly. She stops fighting and wraps her arms around me, too, grabbing the back of my shirt. She cries, her whole body shaking. I see Walter sitting on a bench with his head down. Tears fall from my face as I hold on to my heart's mother like she is keeping my feet on the ground.

Chapter Thirty

I lift my head off of the steering wheel and look out my windshield. My mind is foggy, and I can't seem to wrap my brain around reality. Rain falls heavy outside and beats against the old truck's metal roof. We've lived in this town for eight years now, and somehow it doesn't feel like home anymore. I wipe my eyes and open Old Blue's door. I'd like to say I've never been here before, but that's a lie I can't tell. I step out onto ground I've stepped onto more times than I can count, but for better reasons. I'm losing my mind, and I've lost my crazy heart. The rain soaks me, but like the inside, my outside is numb, too. Music flows through the opened door of the small-town bar, and like a zombie, I walk inside. Sweet guitar strings are strummed, but all I hear is the ringing in my ears. I take a seat on the barstool as Banner walks over.

"Heavy rain tonight," he says, sliding a napkin in front of me. I look at the napkin and then up at his face.

"Jack—straight up."

He narrows his eyes, but doesn't question me. I watch him as he reaches up to grab a shot glass. Looking down at my hands, I run a finger over the dried blood that covers my palm. Water drops from the tip of my baseball hat, and my eyes

shut for a brief moment. Memories flood my mind–
–blonde curls and baby blue eyes. Painful moments and a lifetime of struggles, but I'd do it all again. I open my eyes and grab the glass in front of me. I toss back the burning liquid and try not to choke on the sadness that threatens to take my life away.

I put the glass down and look up when Banner asks, "Another?" I nod and my hand shakes as I bring it to my greedy mouth. "You okay, Cash? Can I get you anything else?" His concern slips between his lips, and my whole body starts to shake. I look up from my shot glass.

"Stolen time," I whisper as my eyes cast downward, and my heart falters. I lift the bottle from the bar and toss some bills onto the countertop. I hear Banner say something, but I don't know what it is nor do I care. I tip the bottle upside down and walk out of the bar, letting the rain drown me and praying the liquor will do just that.

*

There's an empty bottle beside my bed. I grab her pillow and hold on to it, scared to cry because I don't want to cover her smell. My eyes close, and I dream of a girl jumping off a bridge. She doesn't land in the water this time, though. She soars. Her arms are spread wide, and she smiles at me. My crazy heart.

*

"Baby," she whispers as I come out of my drunken sleep. I wake, but I'm the only one here. Rolling over, I cast my eyes to the ceiling as my chest quivers, and I sob like a small child.

*

Standing far away from the funeral Debbie planned, I hear the words the preacher says, and I direct my sight on my little girl holding Leigh's hand. I grip on to the bottle and tip it up before walking away.

*

Rolling off the couch, I fall onto the floor and look up at the ceiling fan going round and round.

"Daddy." I hear and look over to see Ellie.

"Are you okay?" she asks. Concern slips from her little lips and that makes me hurt more.

"No, baby. Daddy isn't okay." Sadness falls down her cheeks, and I sit up and hold my arms out for her to come to me. She does, and I grip her tight as we both cry.

*

Days go by and soon weeks do, too. I'm a wreck, but I pretend to be okay. I drink every night so I can fall asleep, and I'm a robot around my daughter who needs me to be strong. I can't, though. I'm emptier than I once was, and more bitter than I've ever been. I'm broken beyond repair. I fool strangers, but my family and close friends know better.

I walk into work with whiskey on my breath. Anne calls me out.

"Go home, Cash. Get better for your daughter. For yourself, for Christ's sake. Don't you know I feel it, too? Don't you know I've been where you are?"

"Anne, the love of your life didn't choose to leave you. Mine did," I spit. After shoving the door to the office open, I reach back and snatch that fucking bell off, tossing it into the rear of my truck and hauling ass to Banner's. He serves me one drink and then tells me he'll drive me home. I argue, but he doesn't listen. I throw a punch, hitting him right in the nose. He pushes me down; I get up and walk out. While I sit in my truck, tears fall down my face as I look at my cracked knuckles.

*

I forget to pick up Little Miss from school, and Leigh stops by. She knocks on the door, and when I open it, she shoves past me.

"Hell, Cash, this house smells horrible. When's the last time you cleaned? Shit, when's the last time you showered?" she asks me.

I sit down on the couch and grab last night's leftover beer from the coffee table. Making a face as the hot liquid goes down, I toss the bottle back onto the table and it bounces off, hitting the floor and rolling to the wall.

"You can't continue like this, Cash. Do you even realize you forgot to pick up Ellie?"

I groan and rub the hair on my jaw. "I fucking know, I'll go get her." Standing on two feet, I lose my balance, and trip over the blanket from the couch that is on the floor. I fall on my face and stay there.

"I've already picked her up. She's going to stay with us for a little while. I'm getting her things."

I push myself up off the floor. "She is not, and you are not. Ellie needs to be home with me, her father," I say, standing upright and picking the blanket up off the floor.

"Oh, really? You mean the one who stays drunk all the time and forgets to pick her up from school? That father? You're a mess, Cash." The disgusted expression on her face doesn't go unnoticed, but I don't give a shit what my wife's best friend thinks. I don't give a shit what any of them think.

"Look, I get it. It was a hard blow for you losing Sara like that. We all loved her, but it's been months now. You have to get your shit together, or you're going to lose that little girl, too!"

"What do you mean lose her?" I ask, tossing the blanket onto the couch.

"I mean someone besides me," she says, lifting her arm and pointing down at herself. "And the rest of your close friends and family are going to notice your downward spiral, and then they are going to call child services. Do you want that to happen?" I don't say anything because the thought of that closes my throat. "I'm getting some of her things. She'll stay with us for a few nights. Clean this goddamn house and take a shower."

*

I sit on my knees at the end of our bed, grabbing a fistful of the sheets with one hand while the other holds my gun. Putting my head down, I sob like a little boy. I drop the gun and replace it with the bottle on the floor, drinking the last bit then standing up. I wobble, and my vision is blurry. I trip over Bear, and everything goes black as my head hits the floor.

*

I wake with Bear licking my face and nudging me with his nose. It's dark out, and I roll over, wincing at the insane amount of pain coming from my head. I stay still, trying to focus, and breathe before I sit all the way up. My eyes land on the clock. It's earlier than it was when I started drinking that bottle. I realize then I've been knocked out all night and half a day. Bear puts his paw on my leg, and I feel so bad. "Poor guy, you probably have to use the bathroom." Hell, between Sara and me, he's gonna go off the deep end, too. I hold on to the wall as I push myself up, grabbing my head and wincing again from the throbbing pain.

"Come on, boy. Let's go," I say, walking slowly. I make it down the stairs, kicking a few empty beer bottles along the way. I walk to the door, and Bear runs out eagerly. Looking around, I see how our once beautiful home now looks like a trash dump, full of beer and whiskey bottles, half-eaten pizza boxes, and takeout cups. I don't even remember the last time I ate a real meal. I used to cook all the time. But now, I live like this.

Bear walks back inside and goes to the box of pizza, sniffing it and looking back at me. "Have at it, boy." He turns back and grabs the pizza out of the box. Holding it down with his front paw, he rips the top layer off with his teeth. He looks at me as he swallows. "The pepperoni and cheese is my favorite, too," I say, taking a seat on the couch. I sigh and look at the picture we had framed of us three on Ellie's birthday.

I look at Sara and shake my head. "What happened, baby? Why did you leave me?" I can't help the tears that spill out, and I inhale a deep breath as Bear comes over and nudges my arm. "You know the sad thing, Bear? I'm jealous that she's the one gone, and she doesn't have to feel all this pain she's left me with." I pet his head as he licks my arm, then run my hand over my face. "Ahh," I call out. "I've got to keep going, and I've got to stop with all these damn tears." I sniff and stand up. "First things first, Bear. We've got to clean this place up so we can bring our girl home." He barks, and I start picking up the beer bottles.

*

Two hours later, all the trash has been picked up, and the floors have been swept and mopped. The kitchen has been cleaned and the clothes and bed sheets washed. I even took down the curtains and washed them, letting them air dry like Sara always did. The ache in my chest is still there, and everything in this house reminds me of her, but I wouldn't change a thing. They say it all happens for a reason, even if it's wrong. I know my wife was sad and tired of hurting. I'm glad she isn't hurting anymore, but I miss her more than words can say. She lost her battle with bipolar depression. Some people don't; some people can live a more normal lifestyle and their medications work. Every person is different, and I hope that one day I can maybe help someone who is suffering like she was and they have a happier ending. But for now, I'm going to go grab a shower, trim my beard, and go get my Little Miss.

*

I pull up to Leigh's house with Bear in the truck with me. Adjusting my hat, I step out, taking a breath and shutting the door behind me after he climbs out, too. I look up when the front door opens and out walks Little Miss. She smiles and takes off running, her Superman cape blowing behind her, her pretty brown curls getting in her way. I open my arms as she jumps up. I twirl her around, hugging her to me as tight as I can.

"Daddy, I missed you so much," her sweet little voice says.

"I missed you more, Little Miss." I open my eyes and see Leigh and Mark standing by the door. I give them a small wave in thank you as Ellie pulls back and looks at me, her blue eyes pretty as ever, just like her mama's.

"Are we going to be okay now, Daddy?" she asks.

"Yes, baby, we're going to be just fine." I kiss her nose. "Come on. I'll let you drive," I say as Bear circles us.

"I don't drive, Daddy!" She laughs.

"Today you do. Right, Bear?" He barks as I open the door for him to jump in. I climb in, too, placing Little Miss on my lap. "Hold on to the wheel, baby girl. Let's go home."

The End

Look out for Ellie's story, or as we know her…Little Miss.

Coming soon! <3

Acknowledgements

As always, I want to thank you, the reader! Thank you for taking a chance on my writing. Thank you to my girls, Crystal, Monica and Julie for always being eager to read my words. Thanks to my family and Paige, my wonderful editor.

Just a little note:

So…I know this story was a heartbreaker, but I'm telling you I had to write it. I researched the hell out of bipolar disorder, also known as manic depression. I looked up real stories of people who suffer from it, and I was seriously so shocked and just had no idea the extent of it all. Some of it was terribly, heartbreaking. I cried a lot while writing this book, so please know most of these words came from my soul, and I hope they crawl into yours.

Thanks so much. Lots of love— Paige P. Horne

Made in the USA
Columbia, SC
18 April 2017